I0782076

THE Choreography *of* CARE

Engaging caregivers in creative expression

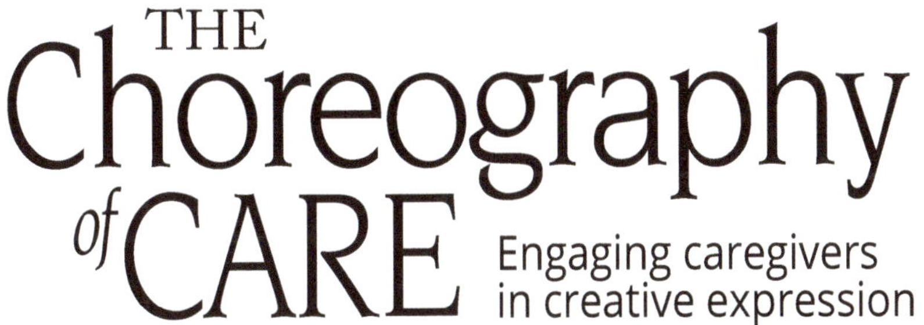

STUART PIMSLER

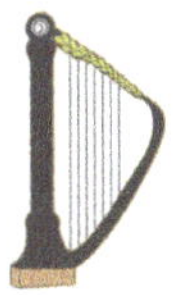

Harp Publishing: The People's Press

Clydesdale, Nova Scotia, Canada

HARP Publishing: The People's Press

216 Clydesdale Road

Clydesdale, Nova Scotia

Canada B2G 2K9

www.harppublishing.ca

Catalogue-in-Publication data is on file with the Library and Archives Canada

ISBN: 978-1-990137-08-2

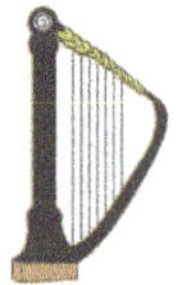

Printed in Canada

Cover photograph: Clark Scott

Graphic design: Cathy Lin

Author portrait: V. Paul Virtucio

In memory of Cecile Pimsler

Praise for *The Choreography of Care*

Stuart Pimsler's touching book illuminates the transformative, healing power of art. *The Choreography of Care* offers poignant revelations about the theater of healthcare and provides fresh approaches for artists as they engage with their communities. The work of Stuart Pimsler and Suzanne Costello asks all of us the important question: how do we consider the role of art in our daily lives?

James Lapine, playwright and director, has won the Tony Award three times for Best Book of a Musical—for *Into the Woods, Falsettos,* and *Passion.* In 1985, Mr. Lapine received the Pulitzer Prize for Drama.

In this wise, compassionate, and insightful book, Stuart Pimsler writes about his twenty-five years of artistic collaboration with health care providers all over the world. Drawing on his own family experience, his life as a dancer and choreographer, scientific research, and the moving testimonies of nurses, doctors, and other healthcare professionals with whom he has worked, Pimsler guides his reader through the revelatory and healing powers the arts bring to medicine, not only for the sick and dying, but just as crucially for those who treat them.

Siri Hustvedt, PhD. Lecturer in psychiatry at Weill Cornell Medical College. Author of *The Shaking Woman* or *A History of My Nerves.*

With writing as fluid and lyrical as a dance, *The Choreography of Care* glides the reader through the personal journey of an artist whose work found unexpected purpose in caring for caregivers. In this captivating and poignant memoir, Stuart Pimsler again demonstrates his prowess as a compelling interdisciplinary maker—weaving autobiography, insight and meaning on the page as he has on the stage for four decades.

Jill Sonke (she, her) Director, Center for Arts in Medicine, University of Florida College of the Arts, and Assistant Director, Shands Arts in Medicine.

Reading *The Choreography of Care* is like sitting in SPDT's own magic circle. As dexterous in his writing as in his dancing, Stuart leads us through the decades of partnering with caregivers to reveal the connection between creative expression and healing. In these profound pages Stuart provides techniques for how we might *all* increase our empathic capacity—which we need now more than ever. By expertly exploring the potent power of movement, touch, and storytelling, Stuart touches us with the power of his own personal story and offers an intimate visceral look at how we might access our full potential through creative expression. The future of healthcare—and of healing—lies within these pages.

Liz Engelman is the Director of Tofte Lake Center and works nationally as a dramaturg on the development of new work.

As a dancer and choreographer, Stuart Pimsler summons entire worlds from his body. His dance theater works incorporate everything from the tradition of Jewish stand-up comedians like his cousin, Red Buttons, to poignant works about love and loss, to deep dives into social and political unrest. Not content with merely taking the show on the road, Pimsler and his partner Suzanne Costello brought their creative methods and theatrical vitality to the field of medicine. Through years of workshops and other interactions with medical professionals and caregivers, Pimsler has created a holistic practice that is revolutionizing the way health care works. This lively and readable book gives readers insight into how movement, storytelling, visual art, and writing can charge the space between healer and patient, caregiver and loved one, individual and community. Philosophers have interrogated the mind-body problem for centuries. Pimsler takes it into the realm of a fluid interplay between the two, and how that dynamism translates to healing.

Linda Shapiro is a choreographer, dance critic and fiction writer.

Contents

Introduction

In 1992, Suzanne Costello, my partner and artistic co-director of Stuart Pimsler Dance & Theater, and I were in Gainesville, Florida, immersed in the privacy of our changing room following a performance of our dance theater work *Swimming to Cecile*. Sophia and Gabe, our children as well as our most ardent fans and critics, were yet to be born and other family members were far away. There was an unexpected knock on our dressing room door, followed by our names recited in a distinctly British accent. A kindly-looking, teary-eyed gentleman greeted us.

"I'm undone. Your work overwhelmed me."

Our new fan was Dr. John Graham-Pole, a pediatric oncologist who directed the children's bone marrow transplant (BMT) unit and had recently co-founded Arts in Medicine (AIM) at Shands Hospital, University of Florida. After introducing himself John invited us to tour his workplace before our departure.

When we arrived at the hospital the following morning, John greeted us in his most distinctive doctor attire. His "uniform" was comprised of a large, colorfully patterned tie, a red bulbous rubber nose tucked away in his pocket, mismatched socks and an ever-present smile. His prior work with Dr. Patch Adams, physician-clown founder of the Gesundheit! Institute, had had its impact. The children were isolated in protective rooms and only visible through single windows. Engaged in activity or asleep, their scalps were starkly hairless as the result of either radiation or chemotherapy treatments. Some looked more fragile than others, with noticeably darkened patches of skin, a common reaction, John told us, from the invasive chemo drugs.

John's diminutive size belied his huge warmth as he strategically donned his red clown nose, pulled up his pants to flash his silly socks, and busted out to sing an English ditty. While he quietly evaluated each child's condition, his compassion and humor lifted their spirits.

I was in awe of his ability to evoke joy and distraction for so many sick children. I struggled to imagine having the emotional, spiritual, and physical capacity to do this kind of work every day. How had John maintained his own health, his own wellness, after caring for and witnessing the loss of hundreds of ill children throughout his lengthy career?

Before leaving his unit, John directed our eyes overhead. Rather than the customary, institutional-white acoustic tiles, the ceiling was checkered with children's paintings: a bouquet of bright red tulips; stick-figure families with arms linked; a girl swimming with turtles; a solitary reaching hand; and multicolored initials enclosed by the outline of a heart.

John eagerly shared the backstory responsible for the ceiling gallery and other creative ventures throughout the hospital. In recent years, along with a committed band of local artists and nurses, he and Mary Rockwood Lane, a nurse-painter, had formed Arts in Medicine (AIM) at Shands. Their mission was to envision new art-based approaches to patient care, the caregiving environment, and the health of caregivers.

Common sense and compassion had inspired the ceiling artwork, an early arts-and-healthcare collaboration. If most patients in the BMT unit spent their days in bed, why not beautify their surroundings? Local visual artists visited each patient weekly, assisting in these aesthetic expressions. Painting a ceiling tile was an opportunity for the patients to gain some small control over an environment they had not chosen to occupy. Creatively engaged, the children and a quickly growing number of adult patients were emboldened by their imaginative powers and distracted from their illnesses. Patients and family members got to witness the overhead installation of their art next to the work of others in the BMT community.

John described other creative explorations he and his colleagues were developing. As an avid writer following in the distinguished tradition of other physician-authors such as William Carlos Williams, W. Somerset Maugham, Anton Chekhov, and Sir Arthur Conan Doyle, John facilitated a writing workshop for caregivers. He also helped to organize a group of musicians who played weekly in the hotel lobby.

And he arranged for a dancer to move and stretch with the children, helping to heal their own bodies in their isolation rooms. (That "dancer-in-residence," Jill Sonke, is now the director of the Center for Arts in Medicine at the University of Florida.)

Before saying goodbye, John surprised us with a request. Would we be willing to work with him and the Shands AIM community? Suzanne and I were both flattered and dumbfounded, not knowing what he expected us to do. We were still reeling from our introduction to John's intense surroundings—and now he was inviting us to become more deeply involved.

What could we offer from our creative process and work as artists that might be of any relevance to healthcare professionals or their patients?

* * * * *

Months later, Suzanne and I found ourselves back on the oncology floor, toting a boombox, an assortment of cassette tapes and CDs, and a shared sense of stage fright. We approached one of the on-duty nurses and asked directions to the room for our workshop. We didn't expect a dance studio but assumed there would be something vaguely similar. We were wrong. The designated area for the workshop was in the center of the oncology floor, adjacent to the nurses' administrative center and the public elevators. Hospital staff, students, patients, and visiting families hurried by in all directions. We asked the arriving participants to help us create a circle using a nearby supply of gurneys to outline it. This was the first of hundreds of circles that Suzanne and I have convened across the globe, with thousands of physicians, nurses, home caregivers, medical students, therapists, hospice staff, social workers, counselors, and others.

This book chronicles how our work has continued to respond to the needs communicated to us by caregivers in professional settings and in homes. It discusses our strategies for bringing creative expression to the caregiver's workplace, as well as the impact art has made on the healing community. These pages speak to the importance of keeping caregivers healthy and offering ideas for their self-care and wellness. Included are specific exercises in movement, theater, writing, visual art, and voice, and directed improvisations for invigorating the practices of healers. Artists of all disciplines will also learn about touchstone issues and techniques for collaborating with the healthcare community.

At the heart of this book is the firm belief, supported by twenty-five years of research and experience, that art has the power to heal the very community entrusted with the public's health.

CHAPTER ONE

He Always Wanted to be a Doctor (A Small Detour)

*A Jewish man with parents alive is a 15-year-old boy
and will remain a 15-year-old boy until they die.*[1]

\- Philip Roth, *Portnoy's Complaint*

I should have known performance would be a big part of my life. My father was a silky-smooth lindy-hopper of extreme grace, effortlessly juggling a lit cigarette from mouth to hand while dancing. My uncle, when inebriated, was celebrated for sipping alcohol from a woman's shoe before breaking out in song. Many family members enjoyed competing for the most laughs as they engaged in wry commentary about a politician, neighbor, or distant cousin who had made a poor choice. However, only one in the family identified as a professional performer. This one exception was my cousin, Aaron Chwatt—aka Red Buttons. For a few years during the 1950s, Red had his own television show, *The Red Buttons Show*, which as a five-year-old I attended with my father.

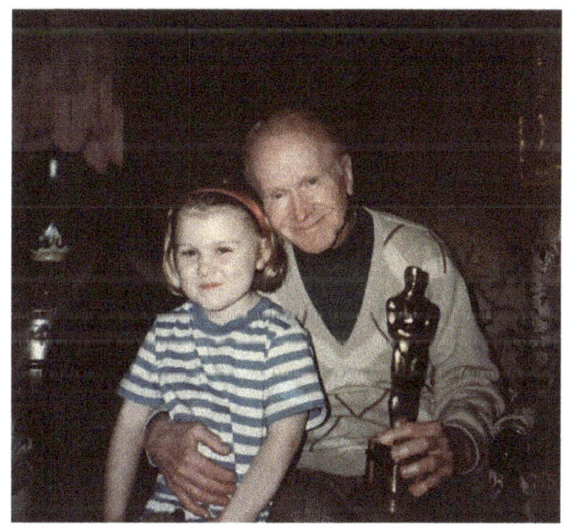

Red Buttons with his Oscar Award
for Best Supporting Actor,
Sayonara (1957), and Sophia Pimsler
Photo Credit: Stuart Pimsler (1997)

Red, a loving fan of his family, included with our tickets a handwritten invitation to come backstage after the show. He welcomed us at his dressing room door wearing a striped knit beanie and offering an up-close belt-out of his iconic "Hey hey, ho ho, strange things are happening." Red's warm welcome made us feel at home in this unfamiliar room filled with mirrors surrounded by metal-caged bulbs, tubes of makeup, and costumes I recognized from the show.

He shared a private space where I witnessed his transition from a grand (five feet, six inches tall) television persona to my sweet, carrot-topped cousin. The magic of this moment, in a space smaller than my bedroom, made me feel as much a VIP as my famous relative.

Not that I was starved for attention—my mother, Cecile, celebrated me daily as her superstar. She lovingly reminisced about my first wellness visits as an infant, recalling my determination to grab hold of the pediatrician's stethoscope as an early sign: "He always wanted to be a doctor." My memory is that Cecile always wanted me to be a doctor. From the moment that I spat out my first sound my mother told me I was brilliant. "Oy, look at him, you are one of a kind." She also assured me I had a face that could stop strangers. She was right about my appearance—it would take years before my considerable Ashkenazic nose morphed from a tragic early childhood deformity to a distinctive character trait. From birth, my Jewish mother loved every flawed part of me. She called me Shimshee or Shimshala (to this day, I still have no idea what influenced the origins of my delectable nickname). Her well-fed Stuie was perfect even when she schlepped me to buy clothes, inquiring, "Where's the husky? He's a husky. Look at him, are you blind, he's a husky."

As I adapted to my mother's mothering, which blended total awe of my alleged smarts with her well-intended remarks about my appearance, I continued to believe that she was also one of a kind. She was a New York City-raised street kid spewing "fuck" in conversations with great conviction. She cried at my bedside when I contracted scarlet fever, fearing I had only hours to live, while she prepared the best chicken soup in the state. My mother was flying over me decades before our culture began debating the pitfalls of helicopter parenting. I loved when she hovered, telling me I would become the best doctor in all of Long Island.

I'm convinced that Dr. Bleiweiss, our family pediatrician, was an early prototype influencing my mother's career aspirations for me. Cecile also had a distant crush on another ruggedly handsome, make-believe healer-actor Vince Edwards. In the weekly television show, *Ben Casey*,

Edwards portrayed a chief neurosurgeon, daring to call out mediocrity at the fictitious County General Hospital. While not as striking a figure as his popular counterpart, our Dr. B. was a meticulous man attired in finely pressed white shirts and tie-it-yourself bow ties.

On one occasion, my mother summoned Dr. B. to our home, concerned about my itching rash. He arrived promptly, toting his handsome black leather bag and amiable demeanor. Upon greeting the doctor, Cecile appeared noticeably distraught, fearing I had the worst (I have inherited my mother's paranoia, as I approach near-terror when my children are ill). My grandmother had just arrived to support my mom's efforts in combating my affliction with a foolproof remedy from the old country: a hearty dose of herring in wine sauce and a toasted *bialy*.[2] Surprised by the doctor's arrival, my grandmother placed the unfinished delicacy under my bed. While certain of herring's curative power, she was uncertain if our doctor would approve of this old-world cure (all of my grandparents were immigrants and had brought many of their remedies from the old country). Upon completing his thorough bedside examination, Dr. Bleiweiss assured all of us that my measles would soon pass. Before departing, the good doctor washed his hands at our kitchen sink, rolled down his sleeves, and asked my guardians if he might have a little taste of the family medicine.

At school, I discovered that my mother's indoctrination, instilling in me a powerful sense of being chosen among "the chosen," was actually a phenomenon shared by many of my Jewish brothers. Who knew that every (or at least every other) Jewish mother of the 1950s believed her son was destined to be a heart surgeon, urologist, psychiatrist, or for the more modest, a pediatrician? How could I distinguish myself as I announced my life's calling? My mother had a plan...

She had already identified the exact tuft of grass to display my medical plaque. Our split-level house with its spacious lawn situated on a large corner lot marked the entrance to Crescent Court (court aka cul-de-sac, aka circle with an opening). "The Court" was a gathering place for stickball and football, and a strategic center for impromptu neighborhood meetings. When I was bitten for the second time by a neighbor's dog, my mother staged a protest in The Court, calling for the animal's permanent removal. I never challenged her reign over The

Court, until the day she revealed a draft of her proposed lawn signage: "Stuart Palmer, M.D." She insisted that after medical school I would change my name because Pimsler was too difficult to pronounce and too Jewish. "You should appeal to everyone."

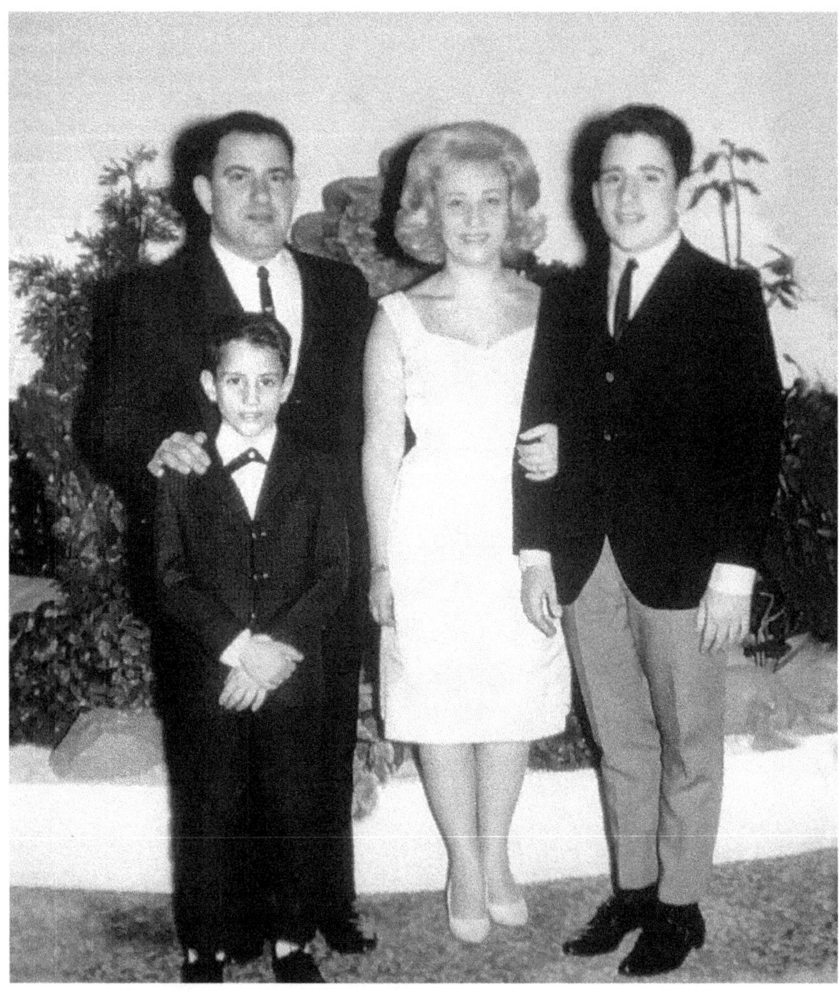

The Pimsler Family
– Randy, Lenny, Cecile, Stuart
Plainview, New York
Photo Credit: Unknown (1962)

I excelled in school although I found the sciences uninspiring. I dared not tell my mom how much biology made me squirm, especially pictures of open, bloody body parts. While my classmates shared our biology teacher's zeal for dissecting frogs, I often took a sick day, doing my best to fake the current disease making its rounds through school. If Mom brought her lips to my forehead and couldn't detect a high temperature, she would immediately make the call to Dr. B. for advice. If she threatened to have the doc make a house call, I would stall his visit with a quick nap and be miraculously cured when I awoke. She was okay with my charade, providing us with some unexpected bonding time and a chance for her to fatten me up a little more with her home cooking.

My dad was a sturdy presence as well. A printer and proud union member, his daily subway commutes were an opportunity to complete the daily *New York Times* crossword puzzle while scraping dried ink from his fingernails. He hoped that I would defy our genetic pool, attain the height and musculature appropriate to a New York Giants middle linebacker, and have a career in sports. It disappointed him when I confided after freshman football that I did not enjoy hitting or being hit by others. I was, however, always ready for him to escort me downstairs to our unfinished basement and instruct me in the art of cha-cha, lindy hop, and merengue. My father, Bernard L. (aka "Lenny," which he said was a better stage name), believed that excelling in athletics and ballroom dancing were mandatory for any adolescent, Jew or Gentile, who had hopes of getting laid. And losing one's virginity as soon as possible was another key component for a healthy life, including the elimination of acne. My father was a naturalist healer ahead of his time.

To help support my eventual medical school expenses, Mom was not content with Dad being the sole breadwinner. She tended to our family finances, and this on-the-job training helped her to secure outside employment. One of her jobs was as a bookkeeper for a plumbing company only a short commute from our house. We lived in Old Bethpage and my mother's job was in Hicksville, a seven-mile drive. "Lenny, if you hadn't made me move from New York City, I could ride the subway to work. Fucking Long Island is so remote, it doesn't even have stagecoaches." Her occasional guilt-filled tirades could not convince my fiscally conservative father to purchase a second car, forcing my mother to carpool with a nearby neighbor.

During one August commute, my mom was the reluctant passenger in our neighbor's seatbelt-less car. As the car edged into Hicksville, a young bicyclist suddenly darted in front. It startled our neighbor who swerved to miss the biker while attempting to brake. Panicked, her foot landed on the gas pedal. Moments later, the automobile crashed at high speed into a tree. It hurtled my mom through the windshield while our neighbor received cuts and bruises. My forty-year-old mother died the next day. I was fifteen and my brother was nine.

My mother's parents, Bessie and Chaim, helped my father organize the seven-day shiva. The Almighty's inexplicable act dumbfounded my religiously orthodox *Zayde* (Yiddish for grandfather). My father, mentor, and guide to all things manly, fainted unexpectedly and repeatedly throughout the seven days. His periodic blackouts were far more devastating than witnessing his tears for the first time. To see my father's robust body go limp and crumble to the floor was shattering. Soon, I copied his behavior,

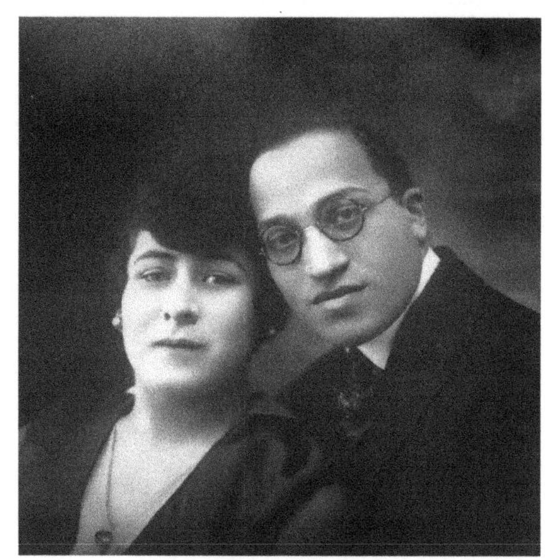

Bessie & Chaim Kaizer
(Author's Maternal Grandparents)
Photo Credit: Unknown

not knowing if I was losing consciousness or just trying to hide. Neither of us could stay down very long, as well-meaning visitors urged us to stand up and be strong for each other. The consolers were many, but no one could give me an answer to my burning question: Why did this happen?

As the week of mourning continued, I became increasingly resentful of visitors to our house. Each day, a new relative or friend would appear, bringing the next offering of Jewish soul food to sustain and comfort our family. As they ate their own food, talked, and joyfully remembered my mom, I became confused. How could they behave as if everything in their lives, in the world, was still the same?

My father tried to keep it together but surely the unresolved grief from the loss of his own mother at an early age was being triggered by the current tragedy. He remarried less than one year later to another single parent with two children who was not equipped to handle the challenges of a reconfigured family. My sorrow was slowly transforming into anger, and I had little patience for another woman who seemed an ill-suited replacement for my mom. With a bag full of guilt for abandoning my younger brother, I left home, living with friends, my grandparents, and eventually my mother's brother and his wife.

As I trekked from one home to the next, I found comfort and solace in books. I would sequester myself in whichever room they assigned me, close the door, and read. An English teacher during my senior high school year provided me with a list of the 100 most important books, which I methodically devoured. Writing continued as another pastime, providing an additional outlet for comfort. The same English teacher, Harvey Grocock (it's true!), encouraged my early literary efforts, hoping that I might pursue more of it in college.

After delivering the graduation commencement speech at Bristol Central High School (the same Bristol, Connecticut, that is home to Lake Compounce, the world's longest-running theme park, and ESPN), I relocated to Lancaster, Pennsylvania for four gloriously expansive years at Franklin & Marshall College. Initially, I tried to honor my mother's wish by majoring in biology, but my innards again balked at the appearance of other innards and their unseemly parts. I sampled three different majors before settling for English.

I followed through on my promise to Mr. Grocock, taking many writing classes, including a favorite in poetry. While a doctor's life was out of the question, I contemplated other possibilities. If I couldn't be a doctor, then maybe my deceased mother would approve of her boychik (a Yiddish expression of endearment for a young man) being the next best thing on the Jewish career ladder—a lawyer. The Catholic University School of Law in Washington, D.C. accepted me, infuriating my zayde. "Why not Temple or Baruch or Yeshiva?"

The congenial exploratory spirit of my undergraduate studies was supplanted by the brusque, adversarial approach of law school. While my law professors demanded the facts of a case, I became consumed by the stories. I wondered about the individual lives that were forever altered by inequitable decisions. Years later I realized that law school, like other parts of my life, could serve as inspirations for art making. One of my first performance works developed as a commentary on an actual legal case filled with human suffering.[3]

Zayde, having recovered from his indignation about my law school choice, looked forward to my emergence as the family's first attorney. I had passed the New York State Bar and Chaim prayed every morning that his motherless grandson would prosper. One day, at the close of his daily prayer ritual, I informed him that my career path had taken a slight detour. Although still early in the day, I suggested that he locate and make ready his bottle of schnapps as we faced off seated at his kitchen table.

"I have given this a lot of thought. I want to be a dancer," I said.

Zayde paused, chugged first schnapps, adjusted yarmulke, cleared his throat, chugged second schnapps, paused.

"Du bist a shmuk," he said. (from the Yiddish—"You are a schmuck")

The rest of my family was also shocked, highly skeptical of my new decision. I had shared little with them about my parallel study of dance during my law school years. Stumbling into Jane Dowd's (first women's sports administrator at Catholic University) dance class had been my healing balm for the cool logic and cumbersome rules of law school. Dancing to the O'Jays "For the Love of Money" in Ms. Dowd's class was the ideal antidote for my Criminal Law professor-priest—attired in his heavenly cassock while lecturing about rape.

I returned to New York City triumphant about my decision to become an artist. Each day I joined other aspiring dance students intent on improving our movement skills. New York City's subways and street-scapes became formidable research platforms as I observed the plenitude of non-verbal theater. Watching pedestrians walk, talk, sit, stand, or even devour a large salted pretzel engaged me at times as much as my dance classes. Was it possible to integrate my different aesthetic predilections for stylized and everyday movement into creating new work? Could I find ways to include my love of writing into the mix? Where could I learn to create moving stories inspired by the everyday?

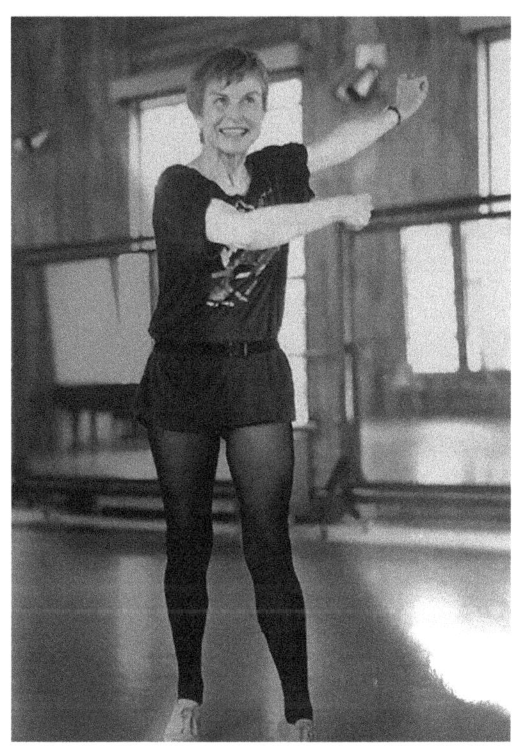

Martha Myers

Photo Credit: American Dance Festival (1988)

I would find the answers to many of my questions away from New York City in the moody, fog-drenched seaport town of New London, Connecticut. Martha Myers greeted me warmly the day I auditioned for the graduate program in dance at Connecticut College. A petite, polite feminist (she was one of the first female news anchors in the U.S.), Martha was also a member of the "early-loss club," having experienced the death of her father at the age of six. I have always wondered if this commonality and our shared need to achieve with the hope of pleasing our deceased parents has been an unspoken bond throughout my relationship with Martha.

My studies with Martha opened me up, facilitating connections between where I came from to the making of art. Martha went beyond critiques of physical mechanics (e.g., focus in the direction of a movement, drop your shoulders, get your leg higher), daring to ask her students what a movement meant to them. Her iconic inquiry, "What's that movement about for you, dear?" inspired me to focus on *why* certain movements or any other staged moments were occurring—to discover how sources of movement can be found in my behavior and that of others. Martha's tenacious coaxing led me to wonder about origins, personal history and its imprint on the body and mind. "How do we respond, rearrange, develop—in a word, choreograph, our experiences?"[4]

Martha's wisdom has continued to shape and inform my artmaking. My life's work in "theater for the heart and mind"[5] has led me to a deeper understanding of my own life while illuminating my connections to others. As an artist, I have been afforded opportunities to better understand how our emotional life is embodied, residing in an intuitive physicality that informs creative expression. In pursuit of my own healing, I have discovered how art can transform loss and sorrow into a courageous beauty. This creative practice, in search of ever-changing perspectives about self, has been my privilege to share with caregivers around the world.

CHAPTER TWO

Into the Gurney Circle

In the magic circle all daemonic powers are loosed.
The mundane realm is excluded, and with it, very often,
the restrictions and proprieties that belong to it.[6]

- Susanne Langer, *The Magic Circle*

With great anticipation and noticeable unease, our first group of caregivers in Gainesville gathered within an impromptu circle. What would we do? Why had John, a revered colleague from this community, invited two artists to work with a group of caregivers from his bone marrow transplant unit and other oncology units? What relevance did our performative work, including *Swimming to Cecile*, have for individuals working in a field where human loss and dire emotional stress were daily occurrences? Did we have anything of value to share? How to begin?

These caregivers were giving up their valuable personal time to try what many of them imagined would take them out of their comfort zone ("Are you really going to make me dance?"). During our pre-workshop planning, Suzanne and I talked about making sure all the participants felt welcomed. In building an atmosphere of trust, we wanted the caregivers to know about us—our backgrounds and goals for working with them. Similarly, we wanted the caregivers' voices to be immediately present as a means for inclusivity and to further illuminate their workplace practices. Introductions seemed like a logical first step.

We asked everyone to tell us their name, number of years in their healthcare field, and a little about their daily responsibilities. We quickly learned there were considerable variations in experience, from first-year practitioners to individuals with over thirty years on the job. John was the only doctor present; most of the participants were nurses and counselors. These introductions were helpful in setting a respectful tone of inclusivity and collegiality. As the circle breathed and opened, Suzanne and I also started to relax and feel more confident about our roles as facilitators. It was time to dive a little deeper. We posed a new question: "Please talk about your inspiration for becoming a caregiver."

The vast majority of responses, then and ever since, mentioned a moment, event, or person as their inspiration. Many caregivers talk about the particular manner in which their mothers held their heads, offering comfort from a fever. Some recall a family physician who always remembered their favorite book or special vacation. Several have spoken about witnessing a first responder care for a victim. Other stories describe aged grandparents at care facilities tended to by a beloved caregiver—individuals who have taken the time to ask questions about a patient's life history. These singularly personal acts of being held, of being helped, of remembering, of being asked, are often the indelible moments that inspire future caregivers.[7]

At the conclusion of this second round of responses, another discernible layer of ease emerged as participants seemed to appreciate, identify with, and support the stories of their colleagues. The structure of the circle encouraged the participants to make eye contact and coaxed an intimacy that coalesced the group. Now it was time for the caregivers, who had just shared with great generosity, to hear from us: How did we become involved in our first arts-and-health endeavor?

We began by admitting that we had never expected to work with professional caregivers. Suzanne shared her experiences related to her elderly parents' health challenges. I talked about the creation of *Swimming to Cecile* as my personal bridge to the realm of loss, a topic ever-present for the caregiver. Ironically, I was uneasy in mentioning this personal connection during this first workshop for Shands caregivers. Would this piece of information from my past sound too pathetic, too self-serving for our workshop? Why was I uncomfortable talking about loss and death publicly? Was it because these caregivers were relative strangers, and I was unprepared to be vulnerable in their presence?

One of my survival mechanisms for getting through personal discomfort in public situations is to explore the humor (sometimes on the dark side) of the moment. Occasionally, I will borrow a joke from my cousin Red or a more contemporary comedian—"I was very close to my Zayde growing up. We did everything together. I'll never forget his last words before he died. 'Are you still holding the ladder?'" Caregivers have taught me to appreciate the relief (at times, bordering on the inappropriate) in gallows humor. Inspiring audience laughter and tears comforts me as a performer and teacher. Talking about anxiety-producing subject matter can help to disperse its discomfort.

During our first venture into the field of arts and health, I told the Shands caregivers about the loss of my mother. I also spoke about how the creation of a performance work in my mother's memory had helped me to grieve and heal. When I had finished my story, a stark silence pervaded our humble circle. Many of the participating caregivers were acknowledging and showing support for me through their facial expressions and forward-reaching postures. I felt relieved, even inspired, to have dared myself to reveal my story of loss. I realized years later that my vulnerability in that moment of discomfort was similar to the fear and anxiety that both caregivers and patients feel in uncertain times.

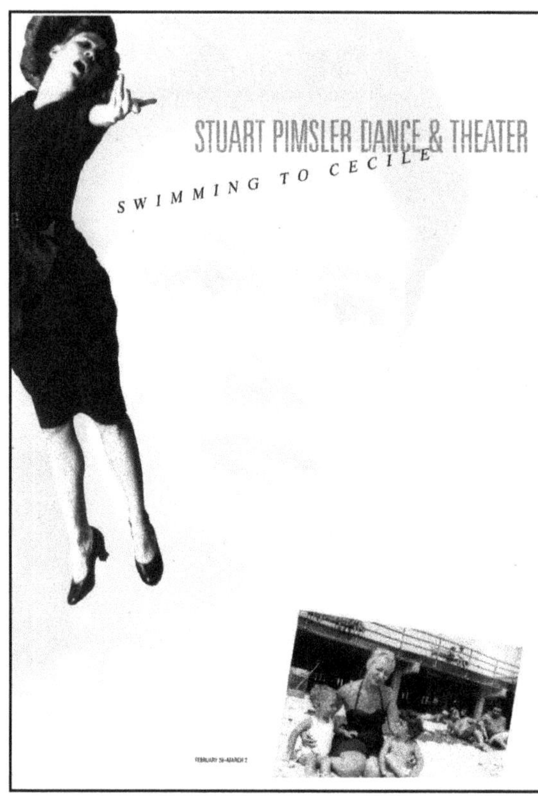

First promotional material for *Swimming to Cecile* (premiered 1988). In 1990, *The Washington Post* said, "In its acknowledgement of loss, its existential questioning and its search for comfort where it can be found, *Swimming to Cecile* is a profoundly moving work."

Graphic Design: Michael Howett

Swimming to Cecile was my creative expression for processing the loss of my mother. During *Cecile's* early rehearsals, I was overwhelmed by an aching sadness. An ardent swimmer, I was inspired by the movement vocabulary of life-saving techniques and swimming strokes. Initially, I was unable to make the metaphoric connection of lap swimming's paradox—a one-mile swim in a pool located me in the same physical location. I was exerting great effort but remained deeply frustrated. Suzanne gently suggested that this enigma might be the link for mourning my mother's death. *Swimming to Cecile* allowed me to access my grief over my mother's passing and provided John, as a member of the audience, with an emotional outlet to remember and mourn the passing of many of his patients. In *Swimming to Cecile*, a solo voice in the dark speaks through a microphone. Her questions and pleading go unanswered.

Where are you?

I don't know where you're hiding.

I just want to talk to you,

For a little while.

A short meeting.

You could tell me what happened.

You could tell me what it's like out there.

What's it like?

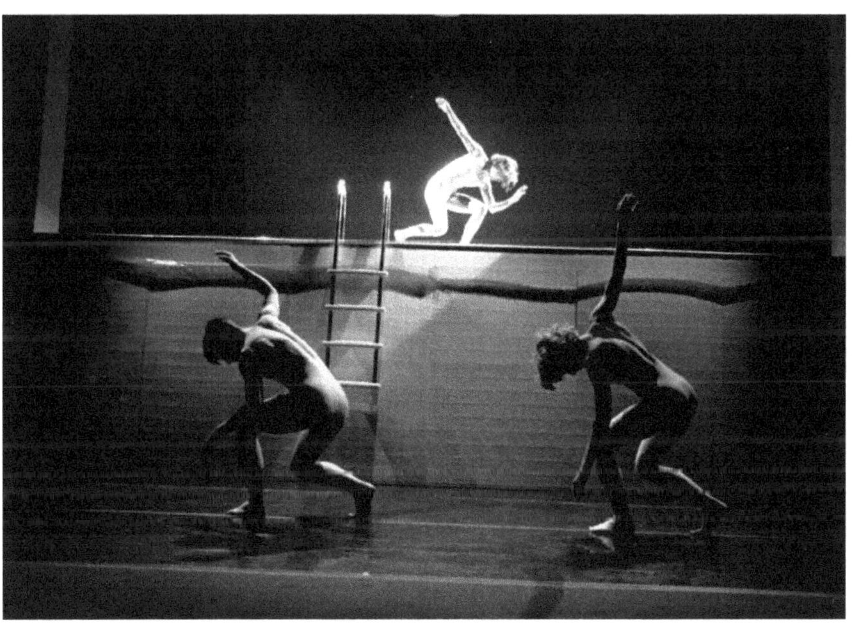

Swimming to Cecile
Photo Credit: Terry Lintner (1988)

Suzanne and I were launched into a new arena of artmaking. We would learn how to facilitate and transform many challenging moments from the caregivers' workplace into personalized moments of creative expression and emotional relief.

CHAPTER THREE

Opening the Doctor's Heart

*He has little to lose and everything to gain by letting
the sick man into his heart.*[8]

- Anatole Broyard, *Intoxicated by my Illness*

Caregivers enter their professions with a heightened empathic capacity, inclined toward helping others. But often when these individuals come to our workshops, they arrive stressed, exhausted, and with a feeling that despite their intentions, they're not able to provide the care they had imagined when they began their careers.

Anatole Broyard was an American writer, literary critic, and distinguished daily book reviewer for the *New York Times*. His own writing had been fascinated with death and dying, including the 1954 short story, "What the cystoscope said," a personal account of his father's last illness and death from cancer. In 1989, Broyard was diagnosed with metastatic prostate cancer himself. Over the following year until his death, he wrote a collection of essays, *Intoxicated by My Illness*. The collection had a ferocity of spirit and opinion inspired by Broyard's courage in recognizing his imminent demise. "A critical illness is like a great permission… It's all right for a threatened man to feel romantic, even crazy, if he likes it."[9]

Even as his cancer ravaged his body, Broyard continued to reflect on his illness through his writing. He claimed that his writing served as a "counterpoint," forcing his illness to go through his character before it could get to him. He wanted to develop a style for his illness and wished for his caregiver to recognize and engage the singularity of his existence and his sickness. "The most important thing for a dying man is to be understood," he pleaded. And with this guiding principle, he became inspired in his final hours to reveal his deep secret to his two adult children. After passing through his life as a white man, Broyard finally confessed to being a Louisiana Creole of mixed-race identity.

His terminal illness had freed him to share those parts of himself he had made invisible.[10]

Perhaps Broyard had wished that his doctor would have known his life secret. In part three of his book, "The patient examines the doctor," he eloquently yearns for his idealized caregiver. In the tradition of family doctors, Broyard hoped for a doctor who would see him and know him rather than only inquiring about his sickness. In being asked about who he was, maybe Broyard would have given himself permission to tell his doctor who he was in its entirety. "The sick man asks far too much…and his doctor may be afraid of making a fool of himself in trying to reply."[11]

From our very first workshop for caregivers at Shands Hospital through to the present, we have asked participants to talk about the challenges that impede their ability to care for patients. We have learned that the impediments can be found in their medical education, and upon graduation, in their workplace conditions.

Physician education is steeped in science and the memorizing of facts, with students barely encouraged to consider the relational aspects of their practice. Students rarely have patient contact until their second year of study, and they get scant practical training in how to perform the walk, the talk, and the listening of a caring human being. Preserving one's humanity as a practitioner is learned on the job and sometimes determined by the student's first mentor. Inadequate role models can leave rookie caregivers feeling overwhelmed as they transition from the classroom to the hospital room. With the particular caregiving environment stressed by client demand and insurance protocols, professional caregivers don't have the requisite time to care for their patients or to dedicate time to their own self-care.

According to many studies, including "Is there hardening of the heart during medical school?,"[12] "The devil is in the third year: a longitudinal study of erosion of empathy in medical school,"[13] and "Empathy decline and its reasons: a systematic review of studies with medical students and residents,"[14] empathy significantly decreases during medical school, particularly in the third year. Potential reasons for the empathy decline include lack of role models, high learning volume, time pressure, hierarchy, cynicism, bureaucracy, and an atrophy of idealism

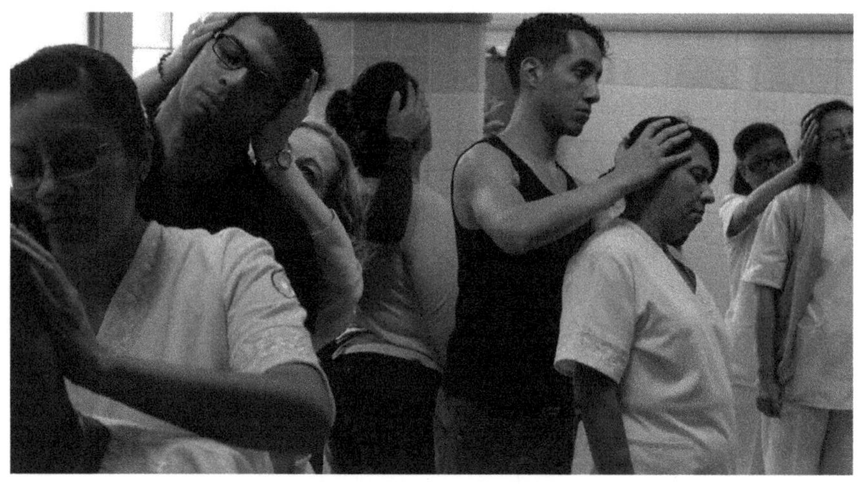

Caring for the Caregiver workshop: Hospital Infantil, Mexico City, Mexico
Photo Credit: Kari Mosel (2013)

during students' socialization. Further, these studies argue that the empathy decline is because of the attitude that medical students are expected to develop, particularly in their third year. "Students embrace particular coping or survival strategies to gain greater control of their emotions and the situation itself, and to avoid professional burnout."[15]

These same studies offer specific remedies for addressing the empathy decline. Each suggested panacea relates to enhanced communication skills with an ability to feel warmth and compassion. How to take the perspective of the patient into account during all aspects of treatment? Is the caregiver willing to walk in the patient's shoes?[16]

* * * * *

In 2011, I was invited to attend a planning meeting at the Wharton Center Institute for Arts and Creativity and Michigan State University's College of Osteopathic Medicine in East Lansing, Michigan. I had done some preliminary research regarding the potential differences between osteopathic and medical school education. Osteopaths and allopathic doctors (traditional medical school) receive similar training, but the former are required to study at least 200 additional hours of hands-on body work/manipulation. Osteopathic education is known for putting more of an emphasis on holistic care, highlighting the value in getting to "know patients as people and carefully considering the value of preventive care and patient education."[17]

The planning meeting attendees included numerous faculty members from the College of Osteopathic Medicine with many years of academic and professional experience as well as the Director of the Wharton Center Institute for Arts and Creativity. The assembled faculty members had earned medical degrees as well as PhDs in Public Health, Masters' degrees in Theology, and Doctorates of Dentistry. Most were still practicing medicine, including one professor who had just returned from volunteer work abroad. After introductions, I facilitated a series of individual writing exercises and discussions, hoping to illuminate some of the challenges the faculty were experiencing. After these preliminary discussions, I asked the planning committee to address the following prompts during group discussions: During their teaching tenures, had they perceived much change in their students' motivations for becoming doctors? What was missing from osteopathic students' education? Was the practice of medicine in the 21st century affecting the current educational landscape?

Each participant spoke eloquently while registering the same theme: the humanity and healing souls of their students were not being nourished. The emphasis on science and technology had minimized those courses and considerations that focused on human relationships. Past doctor-patient relationship courses covered interviewing techniques, emphasizing a patient's medical history. Students were typically evaluated from videotape recordings. Evaluations were based on a checklist of requisite questions asked by the student interviewer, as opposed to any assessments relating to the student's demeanor—facial expression, gaze, posture, etc. Again, students were memorizing skills for patient evaluations based on scientific protocols prescribed in textbooks and classes. But many lacked personal self-awareness of how to interact with a person seeking their advice and care.

These planning sessions informed our new program—*Transforming the Doctor-Patient Relationship*—commissioned by Michigan State University. Six areas of concern emerged from the planning and became the focus of our eight-year relationship with the MSU College of Osteopathy.

- How important is it for the professional caregiver to better understand themselves as a primary vehicle for understanding their patients?

- What are the necessary ingredients (and the importance) for illuminating the patients' entire story that goes beyond their medical chart?

- How do we find the balance between the scientific vs. spiritual relationship with our patients?

- How do we, as professional caregivers in the 21st century, maintain our humanity in a system that often emphasizes the "bottom line"?

- Is there room in our profession to admit that we are flawed and limited, or even to apologize, without worrying about a lawsuit?

- How can the infusion of the arts help to address these issues and provide an illuminating experience for future practitioners?

In addressing these topics through our programs, healthcare students and practitioners continue to make new discoveries about how to relate to their patients. Participants have spoken about the importance of watching individuals as they speak and asking about different aspects of their lives. (Annual healthcare appointments with my physician always begin with each of us providing updates about our families, work and travel highlights.) Being eye-level, resisting interruptions, and allowing for silence are other rudimentary techniques inspired by our work. Caregivers tell us how they are trained to study patients for treatment but often lack skills for observing and talking to an individual.

Our workshops are filled with storytelling that flows from preliminary introductions to early recollections about being cared for. As workshops conclude (particularly those with a large number of attendees), participants will quite often confess to remembering a colleague's story more than their name. Walking in the patient's shoes asks the caregiver to invite the entire individual, body and soul, into a relationship—to take the patient where they are.

During a break at a 2013 symposium/workshop, *Transforming the Doctor-Patient Relationship*, for first and second-year students and faculty at Michigan State University's College of Osteopathic Medicine, a participating student eagerly approached me. He was exuberant in expressing his appreciation for the work we had covered in the first day. Like many of his colleagues he spoke of the extreme rigor of his studies, primarily focused on memorization and "hard science." He felt renewed and enriched to have focused inwards and remembered why he had become a doctor. And with the utmost earnestness of self-discovery, he continued, "these exercises you have engaged us in have made me realize how relational the practice of medicine is. I never really knew that before today." In this moment I felt both professionally gratified and personally horrified. Here was yet another confirmation of a huge omission in medical training. While students were learning about the physical aspects of what made the human tick, the very core of the doctor-patient relationship was being forgotten.

* * * * *

After graduation, workplace realities provoke the heart and soul of the caregiver. Illness, human suffering, and death are the everyday conditions of the caregiver's workplace. Some attention has been given to the severity and tragedy of war veterans suffering from PTSD, and yet, "studies confirm that caregivers play host to a high level of compassion fatigue."[18]

All aspects of caregiving, from the extreme, life-threatening environments of pediatric bone marrow transplant units and emergency rooms to the everyday duress of intensive care units and addiction clinics to the life cycle realities of elder and hospice care, eventually imprint the caregiver's day-to-day life. This emotional residue can weigh down even the most resilient of caregivers. Mother Teresa understood compassion fatigue. She wrote in her plan to her superiors that it was mandatory for her nuns to take an entire year off from their duties every four or five years to allow them to heal from the effects of their caregiving work.[19]

It's no coincidence that while the healthcare professions are projected to be the fastest growing industry in America, doctors and nurses are leaving it at higher rates than almost any other. A survey of nearly 7,000 U.S. physicians, published by the Mayo Clinic Proceedings, reported that one in fifty planned to leave medicine altogether in the next two years, while one in five planned to reduce clinical hours over the next year. Reasons offered for the rise in professional burnout included too many bureaucratic tasks and hours at work, increased computerization of practice, and "just feeling like a cog in a wheel."[20] Burned-out doctors are more likely to make medical errors, work less efficiently, and refer their patients to other caregivers, increasing the overall complexity (and with it, the cost) of care.

"I've learned that we can't treat the patient as a whole person because we are not allowed, as physicians, to be whole people."[21]
- *Transforming the Doctor-Patient Relationship* Workshop Participant

Much has changed since the days when family doctors treated generations of families—entire communities, really—in their homes. Sitting at the bedside in a patient's home provided a broader context for informing the relationship between patient and healer. Beyond dietary preferences, physician house calls afforded caregivers an array of lifestyle information: living conditions, family makeup, cultural alignments, lifestyle interests, and other input related to their patient's wellness. Today, with a hyper-focus on the biology of disease and its concomitant regimen of drugs, surgery, and technological expertise, medicine has strayed from its core context. Yes, biological research and discoveries have dramatically extended life expectancy and eased suffering, but we have left something out.

What's missing? It's more than just enjoying a plate of herring in a patient's home. It's the encounter. The relationship between doctor and patient is overlooked. In Anatole Broyard's plea for a humanistic healer was a prescient distinction, finally being made today, between the concepts of illness and disease—a distinction more profound than mere wordplay. "Illness means what the patient feels when he goes to the doctor and disease means what he has on the way home from the doctor."[22] An organ has a disease but a person carries an illness.

Broyard's hope of connecting to a healer willing to venture beyond the flesh, bones, and marrow of patients—to enter their emotional lives—has emerged as a critical aspect of contemporary medicine. The science of modern medicine has traditionally linked disease to the abnormalities of structure and function of body organs and systems. It filters the medical model of ill health through the recurring, universal identities of diseases such as diabetes and tuberculosis. On the other hand, the concept of illness embraces factors beyond physical and biochemical measurements such as weight, height, blood pressure, heart rate, and other markers. Personal, social, and cultural factors are considered as vital to a diagnosis as the pro forma medical chart.

The distinction between disease and illness carries with it a critical shift in the perspective of viewing ill health. Disease places the responsibility of diagnosis primarily on the doctor as the expert trained to analyze the biologic. Illness is viewed with a nod to patients' perspective on their own health. Meaning and diagnostic potential derive from the patient's experience. Illness includes the subjective response of patients to their condition and how behavior and relationships are impacted by changes in health.

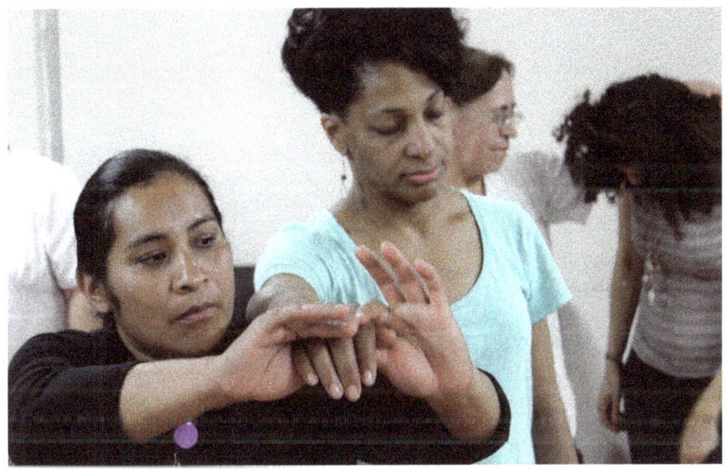

Caring for the Caregiver workshop: Xoco Hospital, Mexico City, Mexico
Photo Credit: Kari Mosel (2013)

This rallying for patient perspective and input has caused doctors to fine-tune, even learn anew, how to engage their patients in a more fully realized, humane relationship. This shift in perspective, while empowering the patient, has also brought doctors increased responsibilities for their own healthcare. The doctor and the patient are expected to pay more attention to their own individual roles in a revised pact of equality for treating illnesses.

Larry Kramer, a Pulitzer Prize nominated playwright and catalyst in the founding of the AIDS Coalition to Unleash Power (ACT UP), dramatically influenced how the public engages with their caregiver.

Kramer was an early and constant critic of the Centers for Disease Control, the National Institute of Health, Memorial Sloan Kettering Hospital in New York City, local politicians, and his own community for refusing to recognize the implications of the AIDS epidemic. As an early AIDS activist, Kramer attended private events and public hearings (e.g., 1986 convening of the Food and Drug Administration), lambasting the government for delaying the approval of new treatments.[23] In *The New Yorker* article "Public nuisance," journalist Michael Specter wrote: "Patients no longer treat their doctors as deities. They scour the Internet, and if they don't like what they hear they shop around."[24] In the same 2002 article, Dr. Anthony Fauci, director of the National Institute of Allergy and Infectious Disease since 1984, is quoted as saying, "In American medicine, there are two eras, before Larry and after Larry."[25]

In the post-Kramer era, doctor-patient partnerships are becoming more common. Michael Millenson, author of *Demanding Medical Excellence: Doctors and Accountability in the Information Age,* calls for replacing the conceptual framework of the "patient-centered model" with a new umbrella called "collaborative health."[26] This new model is urged in response to the technological, economic, and social changes impacting the healthcare community. Examples of these new doctor-patient collaborations are present throughout the world.

The European League Against Rheumatism, a collaborative organization of doctors and patients in 25 countries, provides specific guidelines for "transforming patients from passive recipients of information and instructions to active participants in the management of their disease."[27] A passionate group of professionals and patients with the hope of transforming the culture of healthcare in America created the Society for Participatory Medicine. And mobile software apps such as Fitbit and Epocrates enable caregivers and patients to collaborate online regarding care and drug interactions.

Patients are talking more, and doctors are listening with an enlivened collaborative spirit. This new relational model fortifies our efforts. However, when the young medical student at the symposium generously thanked me, it was an indicator that there was more to do. Could our work contribute to amplifying the communicative potential between the healer and the patient?

CHAPTER FOUR

Why Move?

*Our sense of self, our sense of others, and the way we
formulate ideas are often shaped by the way we move,
by the way we expect others to move.*[28]

\- Raffi Khatchadourian

The human body is a powerful source of communication. Non-verbal cueing informs our decision-making. We often draw conclusions about people based on their postures and gestures. American author and psychiatrist Judith Orloff cites research showing that words account for only seven percent of how we communicate, whereas our body language (55 percent) and tone of voice (38 percent) represent the rest.[29]

People-watching at an airport, concert, grocery store, busy street, or any public gathering spot (including a doctor's office) can be an engaging source of performance. There is much to be read from each tableau—solo travelers, couples, families, groups such as teams or clubs—without listening to a single spoken word. Visual analyses of body postures and body motion serve as an initial filter for a vast array of social judgments. As we observe the movements and actions of those around us, entire stories unfold. Moments of free public theater occur daily.

Contrast two soloists, one with a long, erect spine and slightly puffed-out chest, seated next to an individual with an inwardly focused gaze and slumped spine. Why does one appear more confident and secure? We may have additional insights as we close in on their specific facial expressions such as pursed lips, clenched jaws, frown lines, or a wide smile. This developing scene is further informed once the two soloists stand and move. The individual with elongated posture has a confident stride as she moves with a directness to her next destination. The slumped figure walks tentatively with feet shuffling, occasionally sneaking a glance behind. In the book *People Watching*, the co-authors comment, "Moreover, body motions and postures convey meaningful psychological information such as social categories, emotional states, intentions and underlying dispositions."[30]

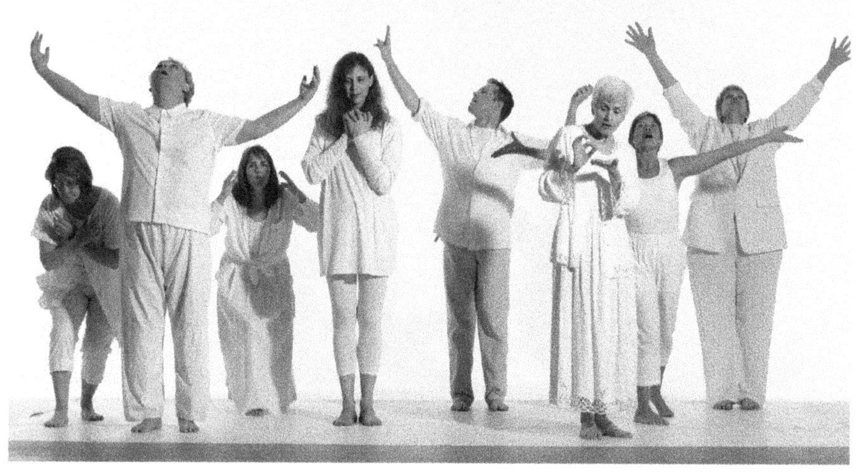

SPDT's *Moving Inquiries* was presented at The Weisman Art Museum, Minneapolis in conjunction with the national exhibit *Hospice: A Photographic Inquiry*
Photo Credit: V. Paul Virtucio (2002)

Consider an initial visit to a caregiver, infused with the patient's anxiety about an unknown diagnosis. This is a first encounter not unlike other initial professional or personal encounters such as a job interview or a date. Both individuals' sensory receptors are fully activated with a heightened awareness of appearance, from physical stature to attire. A doctor who greets a patient with arms across her chest, downward focus, and disinterested vocal expression might serve up a certain patient experience different from that of another doctor offering a simple handshake, imbued with strength and comfort, accompanied by a warm, open gaze. Often, the very first read of anyone, including caregivers, can set the tone and direction of any potential relationship.[31]

Our movement vernacular is as habitual as other forms of expression. Those familiar with our daily patterns may have a keen sense of us before we utter a word. Life partners can articulate their companion's temperaments by observing telltale postures and gestures. Anthropologist and dance scholar Judith Lynne Hanna says, "We think not just with our brains but in collaboration with our bodies because thought processes are in part based on physical experiences of the body."[32] Brain research is proving that movement—the muscular response to an action—is not merely a physical and emotional response. As a form of embodied cognition, movement is one of many senses sent to the brain as a first form of information.[33] At a sensory level, the specificity of our movements provides clues to who we are.

Do caregivers need to enroll in the next series of classes offered by the nearest ballet, modern dance, hip-hop, or ballroom instructor? Maybe not. But there is much for caregivers to learn about themselves as they discover their predilections for nonverbal behavior. Author Kimerer L. LaMothe says, "As this sensory awareness of our movement-making grows, we have within ourselves an instrument of discernment capable of guiding us to assess the value and benefits, the pain and pleasure, of making one movement rather than another."[34]

More and more research focuses on the relational aspects between caregiver and patient, including the caregiver's empathic capacity. Patients heal when doctors reveal to them some readable emotional response. Our projects with caregivers bring attention to vocal tonalities, the non-verbal signaling of postures and gestures, and the language of diagnosis; in each of these communicative realms, the caregiver transmits significant cues that can frame the emotional dynamic between themselves and their patients.

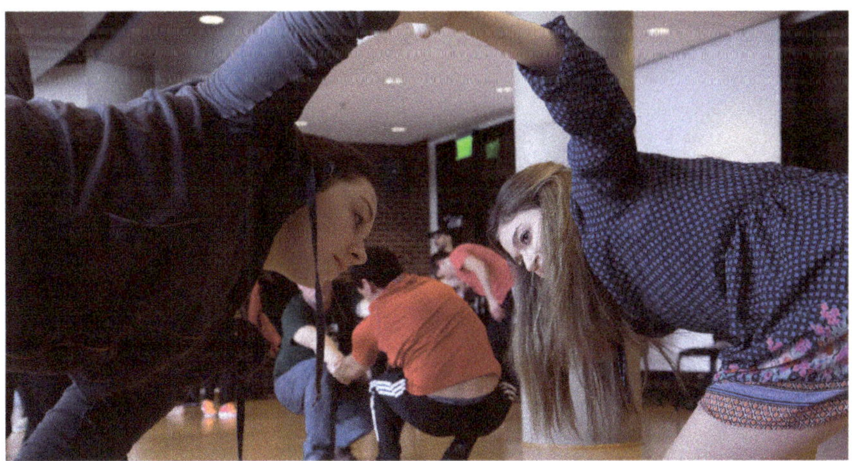

Transforming the Doctor-Patient Relationship
Michigan State University, East Lansing, Michigan
Photo Credit: Stuart Pimsler (2017)

Our creative techniques blend moving, acting, writing, singing, and drawing, focused on the motivation for making specific creative choices. We are less concerned with the "technical how" of a particular artistic response than with the why.

Why is he or isn't he engaging with a specific exercise? Why are some participants finding difficulty looking into the eyes of a passerby while walking through the room? Does one feel more comfortable holding another, versus being held? Is she reluctant to contribute in a group setting? Such self-reflective prompting is woven throughout our undertakings without judgment.

As part of our exercise, *Sabi* (fully described in Chapter 5), we invite participants to work with a partner. One individual with eyes closed is asked to trust their open-eyed partner to guide them through the room. Before moving through the space, we facilitate sequential movements—one person will hold and move the hand, arms, shoulders and head of their partner. Along the way, we encourage both individuals to trust each other. We ask the guide to apply clear nonverbal signals that welcome the weighted release of their partner's limbs and head. We ask the eyes-shut partner to reflect on which parts of their body they are able to release—yielding to another. At the end of *Sabi*, we fine tune the focus, asking participants to consider their experience of having their head held.

- Were you able to let your head be held by another, feeling its weight in your partner's hands? (letting go)

- What did you experience/feel if you were not able to release your head to your partner? (holding on)

- Did you try to help your partner by assisting them in moving your own head? (helping)

During the group debrief of *Sabi*, we ask participants to consider their experience, uncovering their preference to *let go, hold on* or *help*. Does their predilection in *Sabi* provide any broader insights for their relational interactions?

Often, work and life habits imbue our behavior with unintended responses. We may sincerely believe that we are conveying a certain feeling while our body language is suggesting something different.

It is difficult to predict how one's inner life will get communicated. One can suggest ways to know oneself but how to express it is the challenge. A caregiver's disconnect from a patient may forestall the establishing of a trusting foundation and potentially impact health outcomes.

We frequently refer to Stuart Pimsler Dance & Theater's "5 INs" while engaging caregivers. The "5 INs" have proven to be valuable tools throughout our careers uncovering how the evolution of our creative practice often parallels the learning of self. Each of the "INs" function as checkpoints for assessing how a caregiver is being present in their practice and in their daily lives. The "5 INs" can illuminate much about daily behavior, patterns and routines—potential sources for fine tuning communication with patients.

SPDT 5 INs

INtention—Are you doing what you set out to do? Are you showing what you feel?

IN the moment—Are you fully present, seeing and listening as the event unfolds?

INside—Is your inner dialogue connecting to your actions?

INtimate—Do you personalize your engagement with others? Are you willing to be as vulnerable as your patient?

INsight—Do you process your relational interactions, allowing them to inform future choices?

Unlike therapists, our creative process strategies do not have specific therapeutic outcomes. As artists our intention is to invite caregivers to access their lives, personally and professionally, through creative exploration. In moving through creative exercises, caregivers are able to suspend and rejuvenate everyday routines while reconsidering their emotional potential. A past workshop participant included in his evaluative remarks, "This program is a great reinforcement to continue 'nudging' the medical system into reclaiming its creative and observant role."

Anna Halprin, a legendary movement artist, developed an entirely new aspect of her work after being diagnosed with cancer. First, she documented her experiences and healing process, *The Five Stages of Healing*, through her solo performance work. She broadened her findings on healing by performing with communities. In 2000, Ms. Halprin authored *Dance as a Healing Art: Returning to Health with Movement and Imagery*. Her book is a guide for understanding the emotional complexities of a health crisis while proposing a methodology for integrating movement into a healthy life.[35] Movement is at the core of her work.

Halprin is careful to point out that her engagement with cancer patients is not necessarily about curing the individual. That may occur, but she makes no claims to being a shaman. Halprin eloquently distinguishes the realm of her work as being healing rather than curing. She operates at many levels, simultaneously addressing physical, mental, and emotional healing.

Halprin's journey is just one example of how artists explore the emotional connectivity of body and mind. And it is at this intersection that a new, vital consideration emerges to inform the doctor-patient relationship. Should we care about what doctors feel? Beyond its humanistic appeal, research proves that the health of caregivers affects their healing skills.[36] Caregivers spend a lifetime taking care of others but sometimes forget to take care of themselves. If the caregiver is not feeling well on a given day, there's a greater likelihood that patients may not get, or sense they are not getting, the best treatment. Our culture has bestowed caregivers with heroic, superhuman qualities while hoping they will always have the answers and the cures. As long as we get better, do we really care if our doctor is sad about the loss of another patient?

With the "opening up" of the caregiver-care receiver relationship, both partners are reevaluating their expectations for the other. As caregivers encourage patients to be more responsible for their own wellness, the public is learning alternative approaches for self-care. The public is demanding that doctors perform differently. Can caregivers become more emotionally articulate in language and expression?

Medicine and the arts are finding common ground in the behavioral arena of this caregiver-care receiver relationship. Artists, trained in techniques of community engagement, are moving caregivers toward new realizations of themselves. In suggesting techniques and tools for connecting physical, emotional, and spiritual wellness, artists are finding new collaborators throughout the healthcare field.

CHAPTER FIVE

Transforming the
Doctor-Patient Relationship

For many patients, the art of medicine is bedside manner, the way the doctor delivers the news rather than the news itself.[37]

- Dr. Alice W. Flaherty

The Introduction and Chapters 1-3 of this book describe our first venture into the field of arts and medicine and offer an overview into the emotional challenges confronted by professional caregivers. We also provided a first look into the critical connection between nonverbal language and its ability to impact the doctor-patient relationship.

In this chapter we will describe the methodology and specific exercises that we have developed and used in our work with caregivers. Our focus includes no data on the correct alignment for a proper plié (ballet terminology, from the French, meaning "to bend") nor tips for improving your cha-cha, lindy hop, or any other popular step. Dance appears in its context as a sequence of movements for communicating with others.

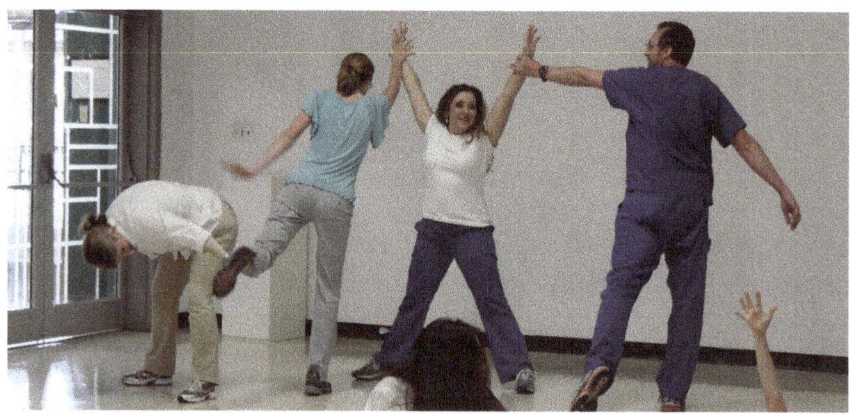

Caring for the Caregiver workshop
University of Kentucky HealthCare, Lexington, Kentucky
Photo Credit: Kari Mosel (2013)

Our movement exercises and the literary, visual, vocal, and theatrical techniques that we use invite caregivers to consider and remember their original impulses for becoming healers, their everyday demeanors and emotional life in relating to their patients, and the importance of caring for themselves throughout their careers. In our own careers, spanning four decades, we have discovered that the communicative power of simple gestures and postures can be as compelling as more complex choreographic patterns. For us, ordinary movement continues to be an important source of uncensored, intimate personal expression.

Beyond self-expression, a growing body of research shows how movement enhances cardiovascular health and brain functioning. Movement exercises improve balance, strength, and coordination, while also lowering blood pressure, reducing cholesterol, and decreasing risks associated with obesity. Movement also exercises the brain, catalyzing the growth of new brain cells (neurogenesis), while aiding in the production of new synapses (synaptic plasticity).[38] John Ratey, an associate professor at Harvard medical school, points to activities that involve learning movement patterns. "The more complex the movements, the more complex the synaptic connections…These circuits are created through movement and can be recruited by other areas and used for thinking."[39]

While benefiting the body and brain, movement also provides an immediate vehicle for stress relief. We encourage caregivers to indulge their kinetic impulses, away from the physical and emotional restraints of computer screens, charts, and life-threatening illnesses. All movement choices are correct, and participants find the pleasure of rediscovering themselves freed up. A room filled with professional caregivers moving expressively through the space is a stark contrast to their daily workplace.

We sequence our work intentionally, volleying back and forth from the verbal to nonverbal. The exercises don't aim to achieve a certain outcome or accomplish a particular feat. They introduce participants to a methodology of creative inquiry and individual expression. Each exercise builds upon an exploration of self-awareness while directing participants to link their findings to the relational aspects of their caregiving practice. The elusive finish line is always about moving toward an enhanced empathic capacity, greater self-care, and a heightened appreciation for practicing the art of care.

We offer a gentle warning to readers before venturing into our "how to's." As artists, our creative process continues as an indelible balance of intellect and intuition. This pursuit of equilibrium often occurs in a single moment. We can tell you about an exercise and describe its sequence, but so much happens along the way that is indescribable, nonverbal. How do we know what a group needs to feel safe and ready to move on to the next exercise? How do we know how to listen and when or how to respond to a charged emotional moment? Make no mistake—intuiting these moments is absolutely vital to the success of the exercises described below. Many of the exercises described in this chapter are best accomplished over a multi-day workshop, as they need appropriate time to accustom participants to our creative process.

PLANNING

Twenty-five years of experience with arts in medicine has taught us that each and every healthcare venue is distinct. The architecture, technology, gurneys, and medical scrubs may be similar but the workplace ecology, from the U.S. to Mexico, hospital to hospice, emergency room to pediatric cancer unit, is always unique. Planning is the critical key for maximizing success in working with caregivers.

Research, dialogue, and ideally a preliminary visit to the actual caregiving workplace are some of the key components of successful planning. Discussions should include a focus on the mission of the healthcare venue, particularly regarding patient care, as well as the specific duties and responsibilities of potential caregiver participants. Emotional stresses can vary based on workplace locales and specializations. For example, oncology units, emergency rooms, and hospices share high occurrences of loss, but each of these locales is quite different regarding expectations for daily care and healing.

Onsite planning provides the obvious advantage of personally observing and assessing the caregivers' daily workplace. What is the *esprit de corps* of the caregivers? Are there any examples of art—paintings on the walls or ceiling, live music in the lobby—in the caregiving venue?

Most importantly, being onsite affords an opportunity to engage face-to-face with organizers and leaders who are inclined toward incorporating the arts into the caregiver's workplace.

My planning sessions with the Michigan State's College of Osteopathic Medicine and Wharton Center's Institute of Art and Creativity (Chapter 3) both extended over two full days. Meeting with faculty and deans provided time to observe, listen, and demonstrate some of the techniques Suzanne and I had developed over the years. I believe that this initial planning meeting set the stage for our successful tenure with Michigan State's College of Osteopathic Medicine from 2011 to 2018. In each of those seven years, we worked with hundreds of osteopathic students and faculty during three-day sessions that included fifteen hours of instruction. To this day, we still receive correspondence from graduates of our program, who speak to how we informed their caregiving approach while continuing to influence their relationships with patients.

RECRUITING

A critical ingredient of planning is understanding the potential population. The demands of caregivers' long shifts, personal life responsibilities, and desires for unscheduled time compete with open calls for workplace training. At Michigan State, I talked extensively with the planners about how to honor and accommodate the students' rigorous schedules. We eventually agreed on a three-day workshop during a public holiday weekend. In other planning sessions, organizational leaders have assisted us in coordinating workshops during regularly scheduled committee meetings or continuing education events. Some organizers have understood the benefits of supporting staff appreciation and enrichment, compensating their caregivers for attending our workshops.

We have learned to craft the marketing language used for publicizing our programs. Different cultures have varying affinities for the art of dance. Some traditions forbid personal touch between genders. We describe our work as a "creative outlet for the stresses"[40] of the caregiver's profession. Movement is included as a technique to be explored, along with writing, voice, and other creative modalities, in our workshop settings. The most compelling recruitment tool is enlisting past participants to convey their experiences to newcomers.

LOCATION

During the planning phase, we spend significant time discussing potential locations for our sessions. Setting up shop (our impromptu studio) in the caregivers' venue offers the comfort and security of familiar surroundings. Caregivers, like other populations who may not be familiar with the process of a creative practice, often express a certain amount of hesitation about participating. In working with us and other artists, caregivers often take a risk as they detour from their everyday routines—informed by hard sciences—into the realm of creative expression. Situating programs in a familiar locale can be another important component in building trust. An environment that is comfortable and safe helps to enhance a spirit of mutual support and cooperation.

During our planning sessions with caregivers, we locate spaces which are:

- Self-contained, restricted from public entry, quiet, clean with access to natural light (We have found carpeted surfaces to be fine).

- Large enough to accommodate a variety of group movement activities.

- Equipped with technology to support sound, video projection, and Wi-Fi access.

- Close to available drinking water.

- Near to restrooms.

- Equipped with chairs for each participant, configured in a circle.

THE MAGIC OF CIRCLES

There is something powerful about circles. Dance historian Curt Sachs and cultural critic Susanne Langer speak much about "the

Reigen" or circle dance as one of the earliest known human dance constructions influenced by "animal ancestors." In these "magic circles" people danced ecstatically to invoke spirits connected with the necessities of life—fertility, birth, death, rain, famine, etc. "In the magic circle all daemonic powers are loosed," says Langer.[41] Similarly, ritual magicians from nearly every culture have created circles to form protective barriers between themselves and all that they summoned. Magic circles are seen as a means for containing and heightening the energy raised during an event or ritual.

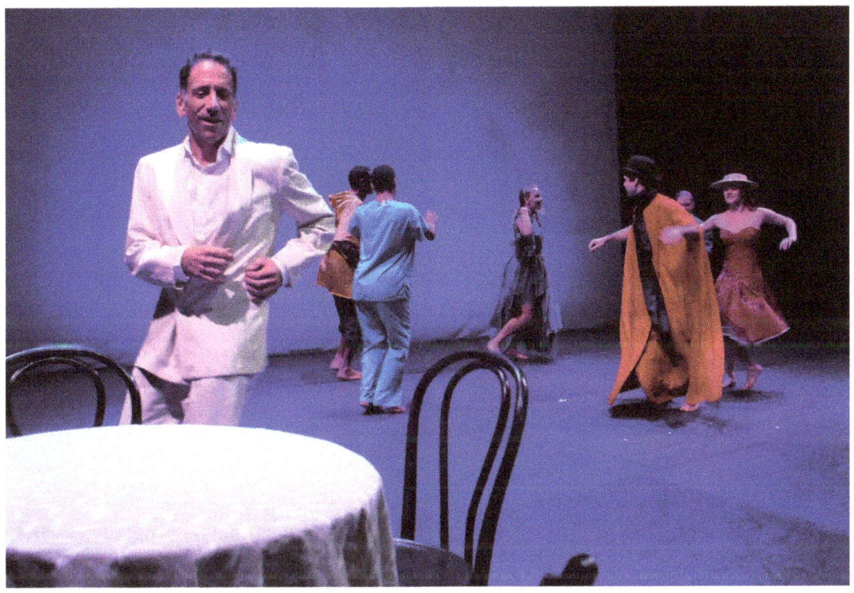

Stuart Pimsler and SPDT company artists in *Undercovers* commissioned by Pathways
Photo Credit: V. Paul Virtucio (2007)

Circles also appear as archetypal forms in every culture, suggesting protection, connection, and community. They have no beginning or end, offering open space for free movement. Rectangles and squares, with their right angles, represent order, rationality, and formality. The casting of a circle enables all participants to see and hear each other without any architectural borders. Everyone faces the equal challenge of deciding how and where to direct their focus as they begin to reveal information about themselves. In the thirty years since the inception of our work with caregivers, whenever Suzanne and I convene group discussions, we always return to the circle.

INTRODUCTIONS

With the circle formed, we ask all participants to introduce themselves by sharing their names, number of years on the job, and a little bit about their job responsibilities. These early introductions help to inform our path going forward. Are doctors participating with nurses, with administrators? Are medical students joined with members of the faculty? Is there a range of seniority and experience?

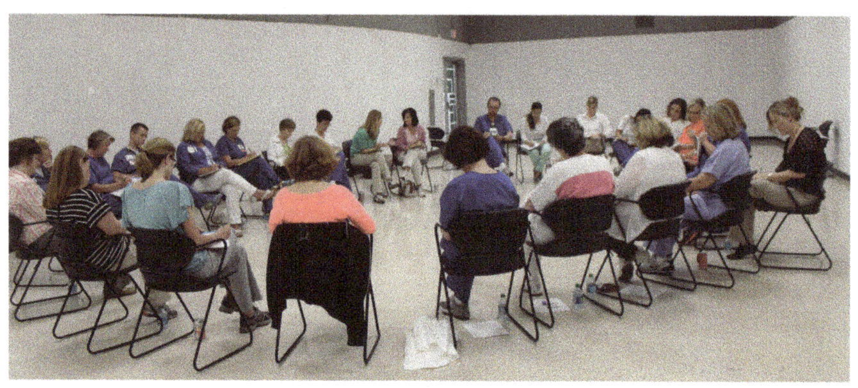

Caring for the Caregiver workshop, UK HealthCare, Lexington, Kentucky
Photo Credit: Kari Mosel (2013)

After Suzanne and I give a brief history of our arts and health endeavors, we invite everyone to talk about their inspiration(s) for deciding to become a caregiver. These first storytelling morsels can set a personal and intimate tone for the entire proceeding. In sharing their individual stories, participants reveal parts of their personal selves beyond their roles as caregivers. Often, these introductions provide new information to colleagues who may have been working closely with each other for many months, even years.

With introductions completed, we ask everyone to reflect on the decision-making process of this first storytelling. How did they feel as they anticipated telling their story? What was considered as stories were edited? Was it difficult to share personal information? "Awkward," "unsure," and "not ready" are common responses. Before moving on, we ask the participants how their feelings might be similar to those of their patients during a first appointment (awkward, unsure, not ready!). This type of prompting becomes a motif throughout the workshop(s)—deducing outcomes from a creative experience and applying them to the caregiver's workplace.

Introductions always include a few ground rules. An extended arm and shaking hand reaching toward the center of the circle is an iconic nonverbal gesture. We invite everyone to follow this childlike gestural lead in affirming a mutual promise: "Anything said here stays here." This mutual commitment to confidentiality supports what hopefully will become the group's mission: to respect one another's voices.

The one spoken goal emphasized throughout the workshop is that participants will dare themselves to learn as much as they can about their own behavioral preferences. The hope is that they'll process this new information about themselves and consider their empathic capacities and relational skills for collaborating with their patients and their colleagues.

This introductory sequence always takes a lot of time. It's important that everyone feels there is enough time to be heard without the pressure of needing to move on. As introductions continue, we often invite group members to mention why they decided to attend the workshop. We have learned that participants' responses to this question can provide moments of levity, signaling that humor is a valuable asset for stress relief. (Yes, these are actual past responses!)

"I was pressured by a hospital administrator with an early termination."

"I was hoping to be taught a section of *The Nutcracker*."

"I couldn't believe that performance artists were going to do a staff-enrichment class for clumsy caregivers."

OUT OF THE CHAIRS

What's next? It's time to change the focus and introduce some nonverbal concepts to be referenced throughout the workshop. This opening exercise can extend beyond an hour depending on group size.

We invite everyone to "freeze" in their chairs, retaining their current postural position. In this frozen moment, we ask everyone to observe the others around the circle. We encourage them to notice the varieties of posture. Do any of the postures provide any clues about how the person might feel about the particular moment? For example, an individual leaning into the circle with a wide-eyed gaze may communicate something different than another who is slumped, leaning away, with arms folded across his chest.

We then ask everyone to stand at the same time. To accomplish this unison moment, everyone needs to see everyone else and find, nonverbally, a mutually-agreed-upon speed to achieve this task. When we're standing, we ask everyone to walk to the chair of someone they just observed. After sitting at the same time in their new chair, we ask them to assume the posture of the person they replaced. We ask them to view themselves in "their posture" now being performed by someone else. As they view their postures on the bodies of others, we invite them to reflect on their own body language.

Beyond the modest adrenaline jolt caused by this surprising request (a dynamic that should be familiar to caregivers), this relatively simple activity is filled with an abundance of skill-building. Observing, listening, and responding are introduced as primary concepts for future discussions. The process also provides an early opportunity to connect a nonverbal exercise to the caregiver's workplace. Caregivers are constantly being scrutinized by the public and their non-verbal language may communicate unintended signals. This exercise emphasizes an important goal and expectation for much of our work: to engage participants in pursuing new insights about their everyday personas.

Getting out of the chairs also inspires another outcome: community building. Everyone is asked to observe their colleagues and stand together. The shared mystery and awkwardness of the exercise creates an early bond. The group may feel somewhat uncomfortable and vulnerable together. Moments of community connection help to reinforce a safe, supportive environment that will hopefully lead to future revelations about self.

MOVE/WALKING THE ROOM

It's time to open the circle and get the chairs out of the way. This offers an early opportunity for creative problem-solving. We ask everyone to move their chair without using their hands. After some titters and giggles, everyone achieves this task, utilizing an array of unanticipated body parts. With the chairs configured on the room's periphery and a mood of playfulness set in motion, we invite everyone to walk.

We direct *Walking the Room* to unfold casually as a welcome change from being seated. Typically, caregivers will take part across a spectrum of involvement from a hesitant, introverted slow pace to an enlivened, wide-eyed, exuberant cadence. Suzanne and I pepper this walking improvisation with periodic directions.

- Are you **seeing** and allowing yourself **to be seen** as you walk?

- How does your focus and walking **change when you approach someone** else?

- What is your walking **preference** at any given moment—fast, casual, tentative, aggressive?

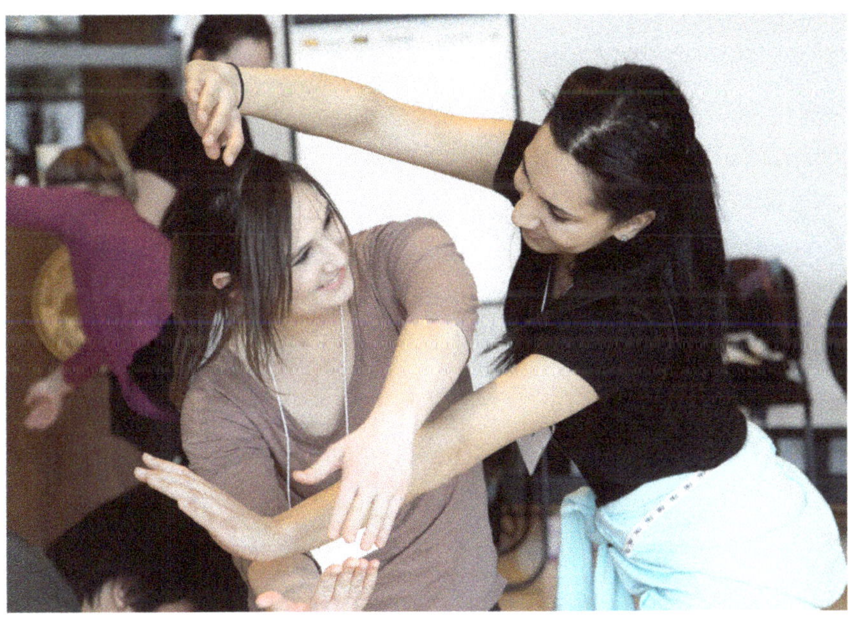

Transforming the Doctor-Patient Relationship
Michigan State University, East Lansing, Michigan
Photo Credit: Kari Mosel (2015)

This exercise becomes increasingly complex as we prompt changes in directions (walk forwards, backwards, sideways), speed (fast, medium, slow, pause), and focus. While continuing to walk, we ask participants to be aware of specific parts of the body. Are their arms or pelvises swaying? We always adjust our directions according to the groups' reluctance or willingness. For example, we might invite everyone to exaggerate particular actions such as large swings of the arms. A wide selection of musical accompaniment is a crucial ingredient for supporting this first movement exercise. Live music is ideal if the budget allows, but recorded music is also fine.

At the conclusion of this walking adventure, lasting from 15 to 30 minutes, we return to our circle and guide feedback. A first query asks them to consider how they felt when they began walking, in contrast to their current emotional state. We might hear "wary, uncomfortable, stiff" or "relieved, even relaxed." We reiterate the concept of seeing by asking them to recall how they were looking at others. Similarly, we ask what they remember about being available for others—for being seen. Were they comfortable or uncomfortable at certain moments, and why? What changed?

The walking exercise provides participants with a first revelation of some behavioral predilections. Immediately, we try to connect the participants' responses to their workplace preferences.

- What is your inclination when you stand and walk—open? withdrawn?

- Do you have any postural preferences, e.g., arms across your chest, arms held behind your back, head tilted?

- As a caregiver, how and when do you look at your patient?

- Is your gaze comforting, compassionate, intimidating, neutral?

- What is your demeanor as a listener—welcoming? judgmental?

During these discussions we emphasize the importance of not placing value on the types of choices made in any given moment. Again, the hope is that all participants will take away new information about how they interact with others. What are their preferences in relating to another human being? The goal of the weekend is not to decide whether introverted or extroverted personalities make better caregivers. If being compassionate is a workplace necessity (and perhaps the most important ingredient in a caregiver's DNA), how will they convey compassion to their patients? If a doctor tells a patient, "I am here to work with you" or "I really care about your health," while not truly looking into their eyes, their words may fall short of the intended meaning.

- *Seeing*

- *Being seen*

- *Availability*

- *Vulnerability*

- *Clarity of communication*

We emphasize these five action states as paramount takeaways at the conclusion of this first exercise. They are referenced repeatedly in much of our work with caregivers.

WRITING EXERCISES

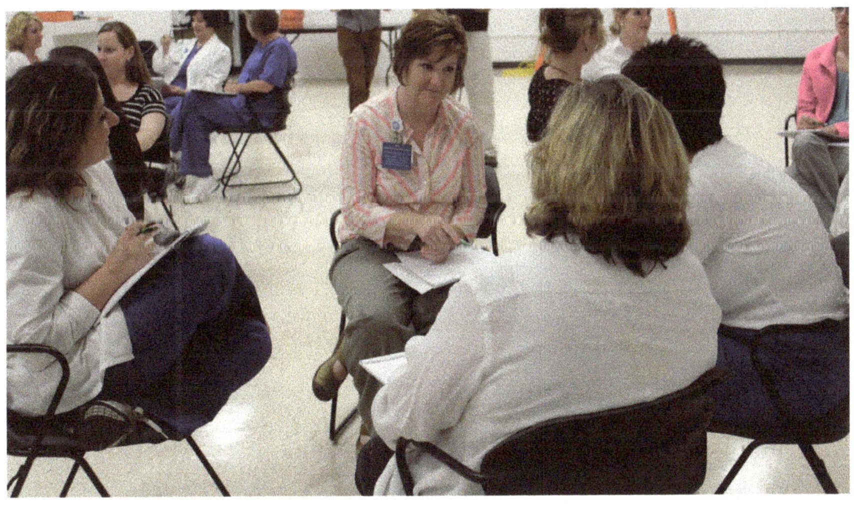

Caring for the Caregiver workshop, UK HealthCare, Lexington, Kentucky
Photo Credit: Kari Mosel (2013)

So far, participants have been engaged in sharing moments of personal history while reflecting on their nonverbal preferences for interacting. A focused writing exercise is suggested next as a contrasting mode for solitary, inward focus. The act of writing allows participants to catch their collective breaths as they regroup into their private selves. What to write about? The specific prompts for these first discussions and writings are contextualized to have meaning for the particular caregivers in the room. Medical and nursing students will have a differing career perspective and requisite needs than veteran healthcare professionals or family caregivers. For example, if we're engaged with a hospital staff, we might invite them to address one achievement and one challenge from their workplace. With hospice staff, we often ask them to talk about a particular patient who continues to live on in their everyday lives.

The following three writing prompts have proved successful for deepening our process with distinct groups of caregivers.

What is your vision for a holistic practice?
(For medical, nursing, and allied health students)

The instructions are to project and describe your vision for a holistic practice. How will you make sure that your practice will treat the whole patient? And how will you implement your vision? Some preliminary cueing might encourage writers to consider patient/client scheduling; types of treatments available; size of staff; healthcare collaborators on staff; waiting room environment; the location, architecture, and neighborhood of their actual facility; targeted population; and amenities such as refreshments, exercise room, library, etc. We discourage everyone from writing generalized mission statements such as "My clinic will be dedicated to treating the entire person, body, mind, and spirit." Everyone can sign off on that statement, but we are looking for the "how to" of it.

We urge participants, as future practitioners, to imagine how they will creatively individualize their treatment of others, and to challenge themselves in creatively thinking how to implement their ideas for a healing practice. When they're finished (15 minutes maximum), each person reads their vision to a partner. This first, formal pairing facilitates a safe structure where feedback and editing can occur. With the fine tuning completed, the group is reconvened, and each participant reads their list aloud. A group scribe records the ideas for a holistic practice on a large pad.

We give everyone an opportunity to add to the list, while considering the possibilities for actualizing their visions. Are there any obstacles preventing them from realizing their goals? When it's completed, we post this list in the room as a first work product. Here are some selected excerpts from past workshops:

- Focus on education, coaching, diet, exercise.

- Provide help to people who are broken. Through small gifts like a wig or massage.

- Rooms for people to stay for a long time.

- It's not about managing your overhead and making as much money as possible. It would be a cash-practice which would free up the middle-man insurance stuff. Charity and pro bono.

- Exercise equipment for patients.

- Visit a patient's house to broaden the wellness context. Can gauge medical treatment informed by what you are seeing.

- Meet people in the community.

- An office surrounded by beautiful scenery - mountains and water.

- I don't want to have to push pills or some kind of product to supplement my income.

We sometimes return to this same writing exercise at the end of a workshop. This affords the participants an opportunity to reassess their first drafts with potentially fresh information. A variation on solo writing is to have small groups come together and collaborate on a joint vision statement.

What are your workplace challenges and successes?
(For professional caregivers)

"I'm spending less and less healing time with my patients" is a common theme heard during our workshops with caregivers. This challenge seems to be prevalent at larger healthcare facilities. Increased patient loads, cost-cutting oversights, testing procedures, and insurance protocols impose daily time constraints on healthcare providers. The initial impulse to individual healing is being constricted by industry standards.

Offering professional caregivers the chance to reflect on workplace challenges can provide an immediate source of emotional relief. It's an opportunity to voice their feelings about a shared frustration: lack of time to "be with" a patient. As they write and read aloud their challenges to colleagues, an opening occurs for group acknowledgment of a common dilemma. By voicing a shared challenge, the group can validate and support each other. This process of validation has often led to suggestions for future support opportunities, both formal and informal.

It's important to offer, at the same moment, a healthful balance in this writing prompt. What are some of your ongoing workplace successes? Healthcare workers engage the public to help them improve or maintain their physical and mental health. Nurses provide an array of critical, hands-on support to facilitate the process of healing. Feeding, bathing, massaging, monitoring, and many other support duties are the often-overlooked daily triumphs of the caregiver. Like challenges, voicing achievements can provide an important opportunity for group support and validation. It can also inspire participants to recall and hold close their decisions to become caregivers and the extreme importance of this life pursuit.

This writing exercise is enriched when participants have a range of experience. Beginning caregivers will often feel reassured as they listen to the experiences and insights of their more tenured colleagues. Meanwhile, the wide-eyed optimism of younger caregivers can provide a much-needed uplift for all in attendance.

Is there a patient that you continue to remember—in your physical and emotional self ?
(For hospice, oncology, and other caregivers)

Loss is a workplace reality for all professional caregivers. John Graham-Pole knew the exact number of children he had served and lost in the bone marrow transplant unit at Shands Hospital. And loss can be felt without death, when caregivers see patients experience a diminution of capacity: erosion of memory; compromised heart; or amputated limb.

How do caregivers grieve and mourn their losses? While individual caregivers may have personal rituals for honoring their patients, the healthcare community does not encourage discussions focused on grief. A Canadian study conducted in 2010-2011 interviewed oncologists with one to thirty years of experience. The study, published in the *Archives of Internal Medicine*, concluded that "not only do doctors experience grief, but the professional taboo on the emotion also has negative consequences for the doctors themselves, as well as for the quality of care they provide."[42] The authors' research discussed the shame felt by oncologists in expressing grief, a sign of being "unprofessional."

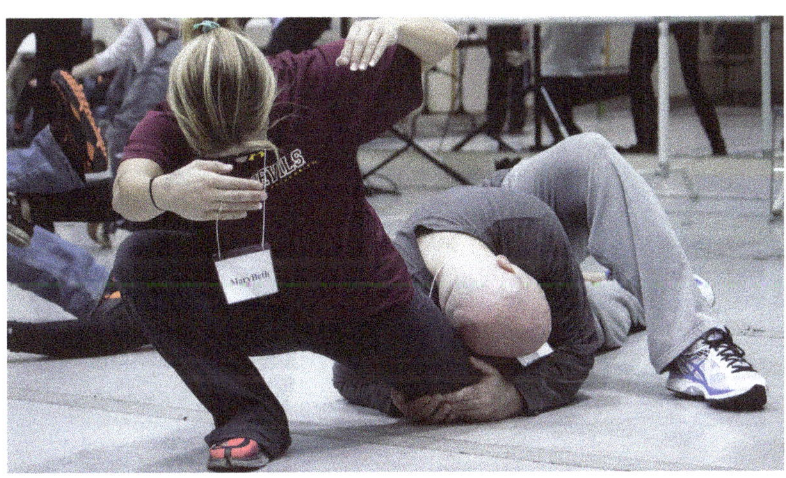

Transforming the Doctor-Patient Relationship
Michigan State University's College of Osteopathic Medicine, East Lansing, Michigan
Photo Credit: Stuart Pimsler (2015)

To maintain their professional veneer, the participating oncologists often found themselves detaching emotionally. However, beneath the detachment were troubling residues of unaddressed emotions. "Participants reported feelings of failure, self-doubt, sadness and powerlessness as part of their grief experience, and a third talked about feelings of guilt, loss of sleep and crying."[43] The study also revealed that patient treatment decisions were being affected as the participating doctors feared the loss of future patients. Aggressive chemotherapy and extensive surgeries were often found to be futile treatments. Further unease with loss impacted the oncologists' ability to talk with their patients about end-of-life decisions and care. "To improve the quality of end-of-life care for patients and their families, we also need to improve the quality of life of their physicians."[44] Providing opportunities to grieve continues to be a missing component of the caregiver's workplace.

Some of our earliest work with caregivers focused on their remembrance of a patient. *Still Life with Rose* (see Chapter 5), a 1996 performance work created for hospice staff in Columbus, Ohio, invited participants to remember a past patient. Their collective memories became the narrative thread for their performance. Our experience with *Still Life with Rose* has continued to inform many of our caregiver activities that focus on grief.

Dr. Naomi Rachel Remen has said, "We burn out not because we don't care but because we don't grieve."[45] The ways in which caregivers deal with a loss can shape their capacity to be present for their future patients. Protecting oneself from loss can distance a caregiver from their practice and personal life. How to replenish one's heart so that there continues to be room left to care?[46]

We invite caregivers to remember a patient they have worked with. We don't specify that the patient under consideration be alive or deceased, only that the caregiver still remembers the patient. Do they recall something they learned from their patient? A memorable saying or phrase? An iconic posture or gesture? With these prompts, we ask participants to write about a particular moment or event that highlights their recollection of the patient. Depending on the time available, we process these writings in a variety of ways from group readings to scene recreations.

In providing a space for remembrance, this writing exercise provides an opportunity to consider grief while being surrounded by other, similarly situated caregivers. It also honors and celebrates both the caregiver's work and the life of the patient being recalled.

INTOXICATED BY MY ILLNESS

In Chapter 2, I cited Anatole Broyard's writing and musing about his search for the ideal doctor. Broyard offers an eloquent confession that speaks to numerous concerns regarding the doctor-patient relationship.[47] Broyard's courageous account leads us from his diagnosis to a despairing acceptance of his changed physical condition. It is the kind of first-person writing that lends itself beautifully to a theatrical monologue.

This is the only time, typically, when Suzanne or I "take to the stage" during our workshops. We perform Broyard's personal account for the group in an improvisational context. We alert the participants that we will be telling them a story based on a patient's experience with his doctor. The story evolves as a plea for help and support that goes unfulfilled. We ask the listeners to make choices about how they want to be with us as they listen. We purposely vary our locations in the room. We might begin far away and eventually move very close to one listener. We might lie down, stand up, try to leave. We're improvising and intuiting each performance moment.

The guidelines for the caregiver audience are purposely broad: listen, feel, and react. The goal of this exercise is to uncover a situation where caregivers are responding in their capacity as attentive, caring human beings as opposed to healthcare professionals. At the conclusion of our performance, we convene a group conversation. Participants typically offer insights about their own behavior as well as observations about their colleagues. The dialogues that follow this exercise serve as a wonderful entrée into the concept of empathic capacity and how we show and share our compassion.

MOVE/WALKING, CROSS-CRAWLING DUETS

Walking the Room is a wonderful exercise to repeat. Its familiarity allows participants to feel more comfortable and confident about being present with themselves and toward each other. It also allows participants to practice fresh information regarding their own nonverbal communication. Are they more aware of walking preferences and their choices for interacting with others? Often, we will next reconvene a group circle and introduce other physical warm-ups. We emphasize that all of these can be useful for many activities or just to get the juices flowing during long hours of sitting.

Beginning with eyes closed and barefoot, we ask everyone to become hyper-aware of how their feet are connecting to the floor. Is the weight evenly distributed throughout their entire foot or are they more forward or back in their stance? With eyes still closed or open (participant choice), we direct them to move their heads in all directions, eventually connecting the directions to one smooth head circle. We encourage them to allow the weight (10-11 pounds) of their heads to stretch them in different directions. The image of "pouring" encourages the head to fall forward as the knees bend. Everyone moves closer to the ground. With the head near the ground and arms extended, we ask everyone to distribute their weight evenly onto hands and knees. Participants are now on all fours, preparing to do what many have not done since infancy—cross crawl.

We describe the mechanics of cross crawling—alternating movement between leading with the right arm/left leg and left arm/right leg. We also mention how cross-lateral movements build bridges between the right and left hemispheres of the brain—enhancing physical coordination and brain activities. Soon everyone is cross crawling through the space, experiencing how good it feels to have their body weight distributed through four points of contact versus the normal two points (standing on our feet). This is another wonderful moment of lighthearted play as we all assume positions reminiscent of our animal ancestors. We evolve from this moment into other warm-up sequences on the ground that might include some familiar yoga poses and positions in which the body is directed to yield its weight. This section concludes with our asking everyone to find a partner, perhaps someone they haven't worked with yet.

While the concept of duets might be more popularly associated with dance, music, and song, the configuration of people in pairs is ever-present. Caregivers constantly collaborate with their patients, and duet exercises allow participants to challenge and deepen their individual boundaries of relational intimacy. It is difficult to avoid eye contact or other behavioral interactions when you are working with one partner, as opposed to walking through a space in a crowd. We begin by telling everyone to face their partner, look at each other and be silent—so very simple and so very disarming. Some of the greatest theater artists of all time, such as Samuel Beckett and Harold Pinter, integrated pauses and silences into their plays, recognizing the power inherent in stillness and unspoken moments. We ask participants to consider situations when moments like these might occur in their healthcare practices, and to project how they can inform those moments with information learned in the workshop.

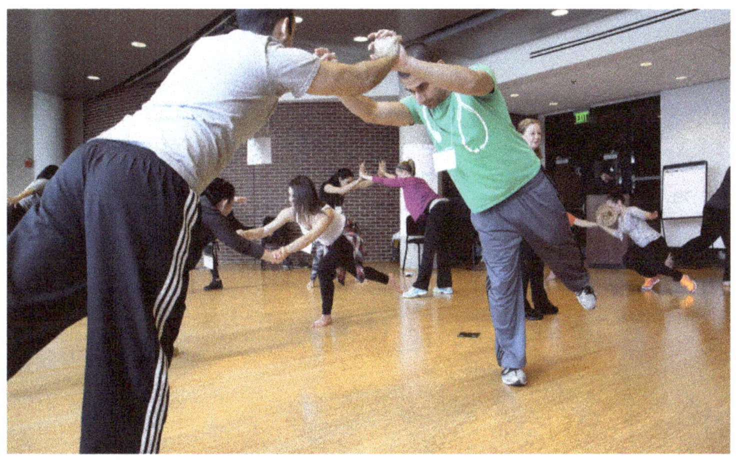

Suzanne Costello leading a *Transforming the Doctor-Patient Relationship* workshop
Michigan State University, East Lansing, Michigan
Photo Credit: Kari Mosel (2016)

As the pairs of participants settle (or try to settle) into each other's gaze, we direct them to mirror each other's movement beginning with the movement of a hand, an arm, both arms, leg, head, torso. The goal is to move together, yielding to any preference that one has for being a leader or a follower. Everyone is working toward a sense of partnering equality, not thinking about who will make the next choice but allowing their immersion in the movement to dictate the journey. We allow enough time for participants to get comfortable with their partners and become engaged in being together.

Next, we ask the duets to again face each other, and this time allow their palms to contact their partner's. With palms touching, we invite them to close their eyes and to provide gentle pressure through the connected palms. They are now moving simultaneously. We eventually direct the duets to find alternative places of contact as they continue to move while connected to each other. Palm contact might lead to arm contact, to backs-to-backs, or heads to foreheads, etc. As they continue, we invite them to play with the possibility of yielding some weight (still being in control) to their partner's touch, taking adequate time to move as fluidly as possible.

Follow-up conversations often focus on how each person progressed in figuring out how to nonverbally co-exist with another person. Relational topics include power (following or leading), comfort or discomfort in silence and stillness, control (bearing and yielding weight), intimacy, and vulnerability. We imagine how these findings might have relevance for their patients/clients and discuss insights that arise for themselves as caregivers.

MAPPING THE PATIENT

Suzanne authored this exercise, which utilizes a bubble map. At the center of the map is a single bubble (circle) to represent the patient/client, with spokes reaching out from it to many other blank bubbles. Participants work individually to fill in the other circles with topic areas that they might find helpful in working with patients. We ask everyone to assume that they already have 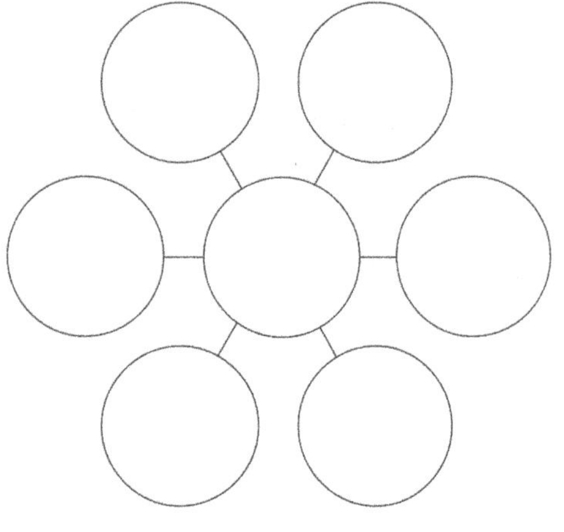 a pro forma medical history and to consider other more personal areas. Economics, family history, diet, home and neighborhood, profession, hobbies, and spiritual life become some broad categories to elaborate upon. When they have completed their individual work, we convene back in the circle and solicit responses that we record on a community bubble sheet. It's important that they support each response with a reason for its inclusion. Also, we ask participants to imagine whether they could feel comfortable inquiring about the topics proposed. Here is an abbreviated list of past responses from this exercise.

- What does the patient want/desire from the appointment?

- Fears or worries. How do they cope with things?

- Are they new to the area? Why are they seeking out a new doctor?

- Who do they feel responsible for? Who do they take care of? And who takes care of them?

- How do they prefer to communicate? Hugs, speech, etc.

- Cultural background. Where are they from?

- Education

- What did they have for breakfast, lunch, and dinner?

- Why do they think they are ill?

- How do they define being healthy?

- What is their opinion about medicine and doctors?

- Are they working? Do they like their work? Is it stressful?

- What do they do that they love?

- Describe relationship with family (describe pets).

- Most important part about their identity.

- How was their childhood? School, abuse, relationships, bullying, etc.

- Living situation.

- Typical week. Is there such a thing?

- Remember the last time they were the happiest.

- Personal safety.

- What is their gender identity?

- What are their thoughts on death?

- Substance abuse.

- Energy level. Motivation to be productive.

Everyone recognizes that many of the deeply personal inquiries from the above list may be inappropriate for a first visit or any future visits.

The exercise is not about trying to create a checklist of new categories for collecting patient insights. Its purpose is to broaden the caregivers' thinking and relational perspective regarding their clients' backgrounds, while reinforcing the idea that wellness is a factor composed of many things beyond clinical procedures and testing.

The physician, author, and educator, Dr. Alice Flaherty, has built a reputation for treating patients whom other doctors have forsaken. Her work combines the skills of a psychiatrist and a neurologist to uncover patients' stories and patterns of behavior that have often been overlooked. Dr. Flaherty brings a heightened sense of empathy to her practice due in part to her own severe emotional struggles following the loss of her twin boys immediately after birth. Through participation in a writer's group, Dr. Flaherty appreciated the healing potential of storytelling in her dual capacities as patient and healer. "In all art, aesthetization opposes the process of anaesthetization that overexposure to suffering can bring."[48]

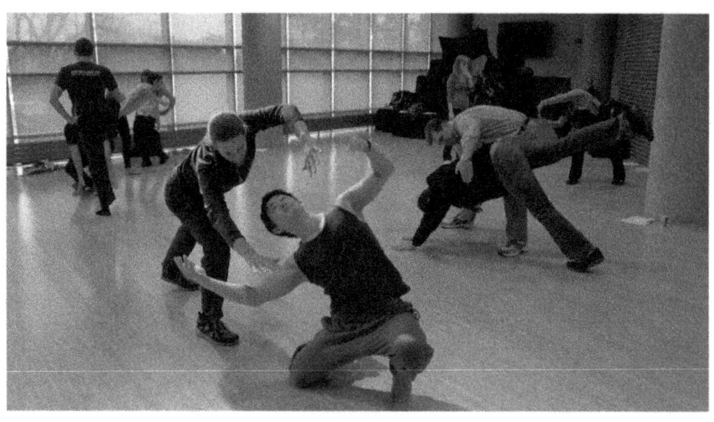

Transforming the Doctor-Patient Relationship
Michigan State University's College of Osteopathic Medicine, East Lansing, Michigan
Photo Credit: Stuart Pimsler (2013)

LANDSCAPES

This exercise begins in a duet form and progresses into large groups (6-10) while the basic structure remains the same. One person assumes a still shape as their partner observes. The observing/moving partner is asked to complement their partner's shape, taking into consideration such concerns as: negative (the empty space surrounding their partner's body); and positive space (their partner's body); feelings evoked by the still shape and decisions relating to whether physical contact might occur. After the duet-landscape is formed, the first person leaves the stillness, observes their partner, and decides on a new shape. This sequence of observing, moving, and stillness continues until the duets begin to move fluidly. Starting as duets enables everyone to become familiar with observing and responding. As the groups become larger, decision-making becomes more complicated, including keeping track of when it's your turn.

Post-*Landscapes* discussions are contextualized around the pragmatic routines of the caregiver. There is much talk about the importance of quality observations and really seeing the patient before doing anything. This can be difficult for caregivers because their personalities, education, and workplaces often stress immediate action. Caregivers are expected to do rounds and complete appointments in a prescribed period. *Landscapes* also introduces a favorite topic for us: entrances and exits. How do caregivers come into the space of their patients? Do they begin talking at the door or wait until they are at the bedside? A caregiver beginning a conversation while handwashing with back turned may cause the patient to feel slighted and irritated: "How can I hear you with the water running?" How can I convey a sense of really being present vs. merely passing through on my way to the next stop? How will I depart from the room? We offer no judgments regarding styles and personal preferences. These discussions are all about highlighting choices while uncovering for the participants their individual patterns for interaction.

HANDSHAKES

It's sometimes easy to overlook traditional conventions of human contact. Handshakes can be the first physical contact most caregivers have with their patients. In *The Handshake: A Gripping History*, author Ella Al-Shamahi writes that handshakes originated millions of years ago, functioning as non-verbal cueing for our closest living relatives— the chimps. Contrary to the notion of the handshake serving as a mere greeting, Ms. Al-Shamahi invites the reader to "appreciate the handshake as a unit of touch (like a hug or kiss)."[49]

This is a seemingly straight-forward activity but filled with much potential nonverbal communication. We split the group in half and have participants form two lines facing each other. One line is asked to close their eyes, and we ask those in the other line to shake the hand of everyone with closed eyes. The line with closed eyes is asked to remember the number of each person shaking their hand (first, second, third, etc.). After everyone has interacted, the closed-eyes "shakees" are asked to stand by the shaker who had the most "compelling" handshake. The outcome is typically unpredictable, although sometimes one hand shaker is surrounded by a clear majority.

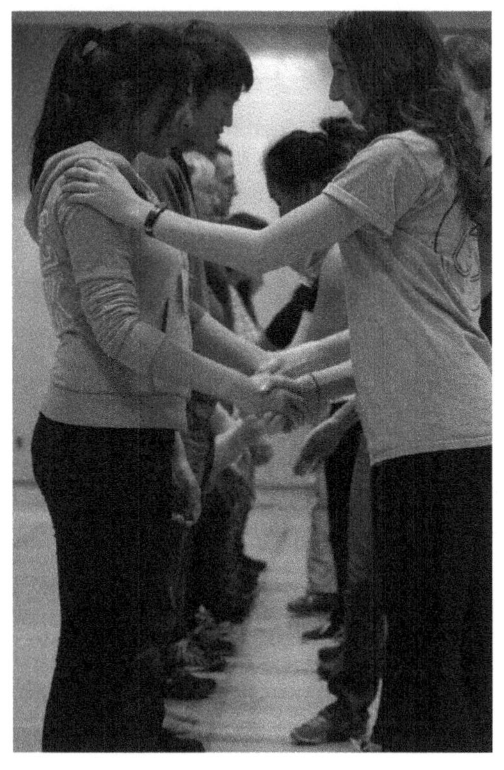

Transforming the Doctor-Patient Relationship
Michigan State University's College of Osteopathic Medicine, East Lansing, Michigan
Photo Credit: Kari Mosel (2015)

The ensuing dialogue focuses on decision-making by the shaker and the physical preferences of the receiver. Participants will typically engage in a diverse range of handshaking choices, paving the way for lively discussions afterwards. How they enter the activity in making first contact, focusing on the person's face or other body locations, single- or double-handed shaking, the time to complete the shake, the amount of pressure exerted by the shaker, and exiting from the physical contact are some recurring topics for group discussions.

As with all of our work, we try to be aware of socio-cultural differences and boundaries regarding physical contact. We preface the weekend and each exercise with safety nets for individuals who may be uncomfortable, or even prohibited from making physical contact or moving (dancing) in public. Similarly, we have also observed how certain cultures often bypass handshakes for more full-bodied first introductions. In the past, our company has worked widely throughout Mexico with artists and caregivers. The handshake ritual, for the most part, always seemed to be replaced by a full-body hug or a kiss on the cheek. This difference in physicality contributed to a very different type of institutional atmosphere at those caregiving venues.

Before continuing, I want to address the new normal confronting all of us due to Covid-19. Loss is a prevailing feeling associated with the current pandemic. Many of the exercises in this book speak to loss and the accompanying (often unexpressed) sense of grief, especially for caregivers. However, at this moment we are being forced to reckon with a new boundary of physical contact—one that is causing us, in many instances, to eliminate human contact while limiting physical proximity. For as long as this new reality is with us, "handshakes" as well as many of the other exercises included in this book will need to be adapted. Artists and caregivers will need to continue in a collaborative spirit to solve the most healthful ways to engage with each other while being cautious about these interactions. One can imagine the possibility of future workshops with participants wearing gloves and masks. Perhaps new discussions and strategies will focus on how to enhance personal interactions while clothed in protective gear. Those senses that remain exposed, particularly vision and hearing, may need to be further scrutinized for their communicative efficacy. Maybe our human touch, even gloved, will emerge invigorated with a heightened awareness.

YES/NO

What about those tough situations when the patient/client is unable to communicate for some reason—introverted, afraid, non-English-speaking, speech-impaired, etc.? How can a caregiver communicate with a minimal amount of verbal language? This is the premise of an exercise where two participants (caregiver and client) can only use two words to communicate: yes and no. We typically have the patient waiting for the caregiver's arrival, which allows the latter to practice entrance and exit techniques. We coach the patient to have a particular pain, condition, or illness that has caused him or her to seek medical advice. It is a first visit, and the caregiver is trying to discern as much as possible about the patient's situation.

This is one of many exercises that evaluates vocal tone and quality as well as facial expression. As with other behavioral elements such as gesture, posture, or walking, vocal expression—what someone sounds like when they speak—can affect the way a caregiver is perceived by the public. Does the voice sound caring or judgmental, friendly or dismissive, attentive or in a rush? By focusing on two words, we encourage the participants to listen to each other's vocal signaling as the impetus for every response. The goal of this exercise is not to learn the full extent of their patient's condition but to practice an expanding repertoire of relational tools.

OFFICE VISIT

This is the most traditional theater exercise that we continue to utilize. It requires two performers to act in a specific scene where each one must improvise in their respective roles as caregiver and patient. While Suzanne works with a caregiver to perform as a caregiver, I will prepare another caregiver to play the part of the patient. Together, the patient and I agree on certain symptoms that they will try to convey to the caregiver. It is important that the patient not be too knowledgeable and articulate about their illness, as one goal is to observe how the attending caregiver will gather information. We direct the patient to create some personal obstacles for the caregiver, causing them to "be in the moment" of problem solving. The patient is also provided with specific character information relating to their personal history. For example, we may ask her to perform the role of a recent immigrant with recurrent, undiagnosed health issues, suffering from acute abdominal pains. The caregiver has the freedom to set up his or her office and receive the patient as s/he desires.

As the duets perform their theatrical roles, other participants serve as the audience. We like to use this exercise when we are doing a series of workshops and participants have become familiar with some behavioral concepts introduced in previous exercises. This exercise, in its heightened complexity, encourages participants to recall takeaways learned about themselves as well as new general awareness. I ask the audience to talk about the caregiver's entrance into the room or the receiving of the patient if they are in their office. We discuss posture, gesture, vocal tone, and expression, as well as the first moment of contact. What is the first word, sentence, or question that the caregiver will speak when meeting a patient for the first time? Where in space will the relationship begin—five feet from a chair or bed? Close up? How close? Will the caregiver stand over the patient, or sit next to them? What is the patient asked before the caregiver enquires about their medical condition? How much personal information is the caregiver willing to offer in hopes of establishing rapport?

Healthcare students do not have many opportunities to practice their relational skills before working with first clients/patients. Tragically, there is a lack of training in human relationship building and in the practice of it for healthcare trainees. Notable exceptions can be found in the training of nurses, social workers and the graduate training of mental health therapists, where "role plays" are typically employed.[50] *Office Visit* goes beyond interviewing techniques that solely focus on diagnosis and treatment. It also offers caregivers the opportunity to be in the role of "cared for" and experience the vulnerability that comes with that.

SELF PORTRAIT

Suzanne first introduced this exercise, and I always fondly recall John Graham-Pole's artful ceilings in his bone marrow transplant unit. Everyone gets a blank piece of paper and colored writing tools of any sort—markers, crayons, pens, etc. Simple instructions—draw a self-portrait with any combination of images, words, symbols, and color. As with performing arts exercises, we encourage participants not to be concerned with technical proficiency and instead create from a place of feeling and abstraction. How do you visually represent yourself? As with all solo activities, whether they be verbal or non-verbal, we always set a time limit for completion. When everyone has completed their portrait, we ask that they be posted somewhere in the room. One by one, the participants take turns providing backstory about their portraits as everyone travels from one portrait to the next. By this time, in extended workshops, the art products from this and previous exercises infuse the atmosphere with powerful remnants of the work being accomplished—a living gallery.

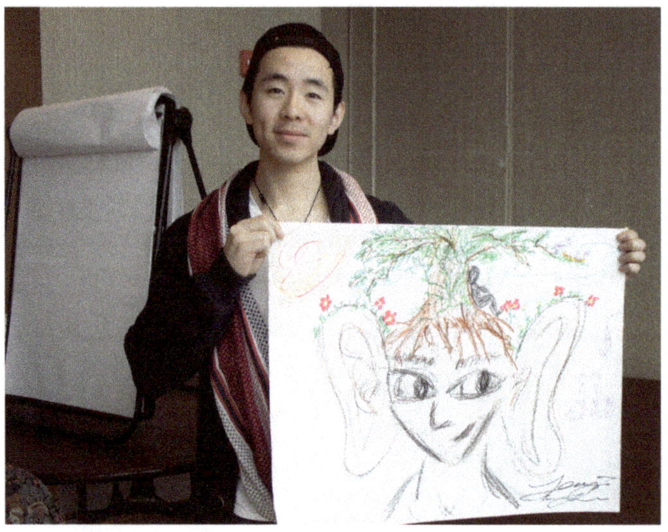

Transforming the Doctor-Patient Relationship
Michigan State University's College of Osteopathic Medicine, East Lansing, Michigan
Photo Credit: Kari Mosel (2015)

This exercise, like others involving individual creativity, is achievable by all and is a great confidence builder. It is another moment of dispelling preconceptions about creative license and who has permission to partake in creative expression. Its self-reflective process inspires another opportunity for participants to go inward, to consider how they are and how they present themselves publicly. It also affirms the power of individual imagination. We suggest the possibility of offering this exercise to patients/clients to determine additional information and for its therapeutic value.

These are some comments illustrating the backstories informing the visual choices made by past caregivers.

- *I drew a mirror because coming here is very different. Looking at other people, I feel different, so I feel like I need to fix myself to fit the normal standard here. Signature in Chinese writing.*

- *I drew the ocean because it is calming. Nature and mountains because there are some good things and some rough things. Sun because I like warm. The stars because our world is bigger than what we think of. I love space. Warm colors.*

- *Earth in the middle, sun. Magnetic field of the earth. Black triangle into a human. Earth is very finite. We are all going to live a certain amount of time, we don't know. To think about myself in this finite place and life. What I want to do is radiate love.*

- *At school, I'm a student. But when I go home out to the lake I feel like a different person. I bought a sailboat. It was a challenge because no one knew how to use it. It's nice to be out in a place when you don't have a connection with anyone. Just me and myself.*

- *I made a plane to travel home. Every time I got sick my mom and I would stay home and cook. I feel like a very open person but I have this box that I don't open up until I really know and trust someone.*

- *The night sky. When I'm stressed out, I will look into the night sky. It's very humbling and it brings me back down to earth. Everyone who has ever lived is on a tiny dot in the Milky Way.*

- *I have a hand for helping others and lips for communication. I went to Michigan and I learned a lot there. Lines to symbolize integrity.*

- *I overthink things a lot. So I drew a lot of things that I liked.*

SABI

(Japanese for rust; as in ripe with experience and insight)

The name for this exercise is the title of a performance piece I created, commissioned by the American Dance Festival (ADF) in 1994. The cast included eleven non-English speaking Japanese dancers and a translator. With new creations, I typically have many ideas for entry points, but until meeting the cast I am never certain as to my final direction. As with all our workshops, I always want to know about my collaborators. I sensed that this might be a challenge with this cast, even with a translator.

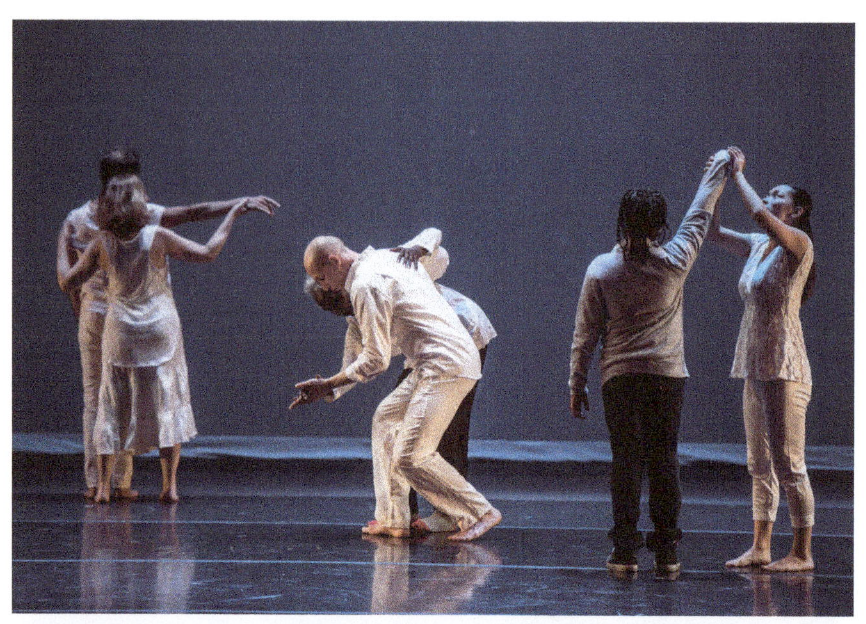

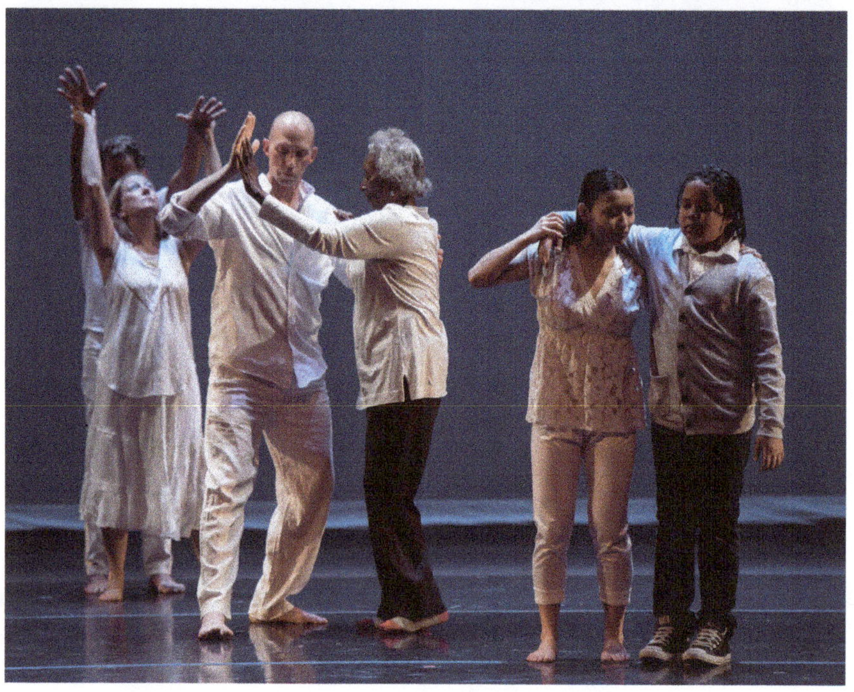

Sabi, University of Alabama at Birmingham Alys Stephens Center, performed by SPDT company artists and audience members.

Photo Credit: Clark Scott (2016)

There are other factors, besides the cast, that influence me when I start something new. I am affected by the location, particularly if I am away from my home. ADF occurs in Durham, North Carolina every summer, when the humid heat of the South can weigh on you like a wet blanket. Moving all day long is a challenge. Our rehearsal studio was an older, white gymnasium on the Duke University campus. There was a running track on the second tier, outlined with full-length picture windows that brought natural light into the space.

My creative process is also deeply influenced by what is taking place in my life. Inevitably, the questions, the irritants, the feelings about some current personal or political event find their way into my creative mix. At the time, two powerful personal events were unfolding in my life. I had recently experienced the death of a dear friend and colleague, Ronald Aiji Kajiwara (elaborated upon in Chapter 5). Near Aiji's passing, Suzanne and I had our first child, Sophia Cecile. My residency at ADF was the first time I had been away from Sophia since her birth, and I was missing her very much.

My longing for Aiji and Sophia was a forceful presence leading me. I imagined them together, sharing certain sensibilities. Both had an innocence and wonderment about their surroundings. Their patient demeanors and quietude lent an air of contentment as each seemed to find pleasure in contemplating the world around them. How would Aiji and Sophia relate to each other in an enlivened state of calm? I conjured up an image of trusted support as I began to rehearse.

I invited the cast of twelve to divide into six duets and place themselves above the gym floor, in front of the windows on the second floor—instant scenic design. A visually arresting image that Aiji would approve of and admire. For some time, I was enthralled with the opening still life of the six couples placed in front of the gym's grand openings to the outside. There was something transcendent, even ethereal, about seeing the performers situated this way. How would I move on from this moment but maintain the essence of this very innocent, caring relationship? I asked one performer in each duet to close their eyes and allow their partner to move them. From this improvisation, I created some very simple movement pathways that eventually brought the performers down the stairs to the gym floor where the dance concluded.

A long back story for such a simple but powerful exercise for healthcare participants. A *Sabi* duet asks one person to close their eyes and the other to look and see their partner, to consider them a living sculpture and notice the physical distinctions that make their partner unique. *Sabi* moves from a place of observation through prompts that direct the open-eyed partner to move select body parts of their partner—hands, arm, head—and eventually escort them through the space. The eyes-closed partner is asked to keep their eyes closed the entire time and allow their partner to take care of them. We always make sure that each partner has an opportunity to be both caregiver and care receiver.

What I enjoyed most about this program was the movement and trust with a partner. And shaking off the notion that "touch is unprofessional."

- Caring for the Caregiver Workshop Participant, Mayo Clinic (2003)

Beyond its relaxing state of voluntary sensory deprivation, *Sabi* invites personal reflection for each role experienced. Do participants prefer having their eyes closed or open, being a mover or being moved, being cared for or caring for? Do they feel more comfortable in one role vs. the other? We suggest this exercise as another metaphor for the caregiving-cared for paradigm. The patient is someone who entrusts, often blindly, the caregiver with their needs and allows themselves to be led into unknown territory. It's important for the caregivers to always remember how vulnerable their patients are in this relationship.

The title *Sabi* recognizes the original cast who helped to make this exercise. The word also refers in Japanese culture to something that has aged well, grown rusty with a sense of aged beauty. The concept *sabi* carries not only the meaning *aged*—"in the sense of ripe with experience and insight and infused with the patina that lends old things their beauty—but also that of tranquility, aloneness, deep solitude."[51]

THE FIRST TIME

Often after *Sabi*, participants are relaxed and feel less guarded. This can be a poignant moment to consider some reflective writing around a memory. Asking participants to remember the first time they were cared for can be a source of very personal reflection and can sometimes serve to further uncover some original motivations for becoming a caregiver. We ask each writer to read their story to a partner who is asked to engage as an active listener. We then direct the listener to respond to the reader with the following three responses: I heard, I wondered, I felt.

This exercise is another foray into empathic listening and responding while affirming for the writer that they were being heard. Like all the exercises that occur in a duet framework, it challenges participants to depend on and trust each other with emotionally charged, intimate material. Along the way, participants continue to assess their own boundaries and willingness to be vulnerable with unfamiliar partners in the same way that patients are configured with their caregiver.

BIG LIFTS

We save the grand finale of physical daring for the last day. By this time, participants have gotten more comfortable with each other and are more ready to venture into bold physical choices. This exercise works well with large groups configured in a circle. Each person takes a turn being in the center of the circle and is directed to lean in any direction. It sometimes helps for the center person to close their eyes. As the center person leans, he or she is supported by the rest of the group, experiencing the sensation of letting go. The exercise continues into a riskier place as the leaning person is eventually lifted off the ground. Much preparation and instruction take place before this occurs, to make sure everyone is protecting their own bodies and understanding how to safely lift their colleagues.

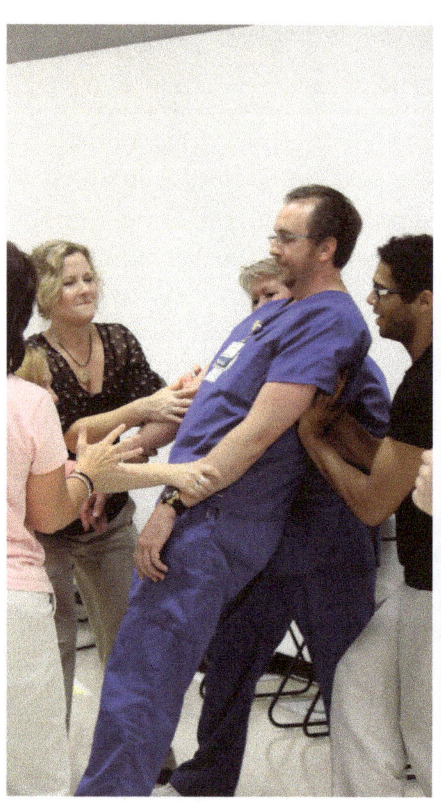

Caring for the Caregiver workshop
UK HealthCare, Lexington, Kentucky
Photo Credit: Kari Mosel (2013)

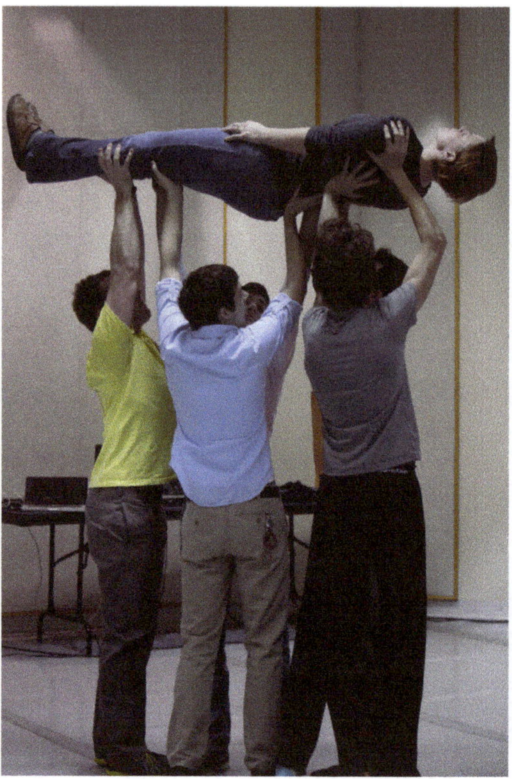

Transforming the Doctor-Patient Relationship
Michigan State University,
College of Osteopathic Medicine,
East Lansing, Michigan
Photo Credit: Kari Mosel (2015)

The discussion that follows processes the exercise's sequencing, inviting participants to reflect on their discoveries from standing to being suspended above the ground. Was it difficult to let themselves be held and supported by others? How did they work together, in a sudden moment with each other? Where was their focus? By this time, observing, listening, and responding spontaneously become repeating motifs. Beyond these concerns, this exercise is a wonderful, fun relief from the more serious introspection of past exercises and provides an impressive opportunity for everyone to be held aloft. It also serves as a poetic segue into a most important group discussion about self-care.

It's comforting for Suzanne and me to know that after these many years we can rely on certain techniques, skills, and strategies that have been successful for working with caregivers. However, as artists, we are constantly researching and imagining new ideas to refresh our work while challenging ourselves to take risks. Please realize that we have tried many exercises in the past that have not been productive, that have even flopped. We've gotten much better at knowing what might be effective, but we sometimes miss. One of the most exhilarating feelings for an artist is to try something (the premiere) and find that it works really well. To take a risk and feel successful provides an incredible feeling of satisfaction and accomplishment.

SELF-CARE

Caregivers are reluctant practitioners of self-care—even during times of less urgency. We offer the following suggestions to inspire discussion, while inviting participants to add to the list. These suggestions span a broad spectrum from private, introspective endeavors to vigorous physical pursuits. The hope is that some of these ideas will spark a fresh interest and become a formal part of the caregivers' self-care practice. We strongly encourage caregivers to schedule self-care as they schedule other things in their lives—so that they actually do it.

Journal

    Take a walk somewhere new, somewhere familiar

Tell a friend about your day's events

    Stretch

    Breathe

Write a short poem...about yourself, about a patient

    Laugh......as much as you can

Get a massage

Bake a cake

Go to a performance

    Write a letter

Sit and listen to music

Cook a great meal

Be in the moment

Ask for help/advice

Exhale

Take a break from the news

Play with a child...of any age

Be spontaneous

Sleep

Play with a pet

Do something you've never done

Dance slowly, or as fast as you can

Spend time in nature

Travel......near and far

Read a book

Notice things around you

Light candles

Take a bath by candlelight

Learn to say No

Watch a movie

Write down your dreams

Close your eyes and listen to your breath

Listen to nothing

Get a pedicure

Leave home without your phone

Buy yourself flowers

Be still and breathe

And...

CLOSING

Previously, I have addressed the time pressures confronted by caregivers to fulfill their educational requirements and on-the-job work demands. In this chapter, much has been said about the importance of providing adequate time for the completion of different exercises—tasks and reflections. As a last group activity, closings should be carefully scheduled to allow time for all voices to be heard.

Whether at the end of a single, two-hour workshop or a multi-day symposium, closings are a time for participants to reflect on their experiences. For many caregivers, being immersed in the personal and often vulnerable process of creative expression may be a new venture. Accessing stories relating to a beloved patient or family member may spur memories filled with unresolved emotions. Sometimes, revisiting these unsettled moments, activated by a workshop encounter, will provide new clarity. Some may comment on the pure joy and freedom they felt in being given permission to move in novel ways. Others might speak to the healing calm or discomfort of being held and supported by their colleagues. It is critical that all participants have time to consider how they have been impacted.

Typically, Suzanne and I will frame closing sessions in an open-ended manner, asking the group to describe some of the takeaways from the work we have done together. We have found that by the time the closing occurs, participants are inclined toward a greater sense of sharing. Listening to each other validates connections made during the workshop, while affirming the inherent benefits of future creative pursuits.

CHAPTER SIX

Still Life with Rose

These days I always read the obituary page first.
I want to see who I know, particularly if it's someone
I haven't seen for a long time. I want to know if it is someone
I have cared for... I do measure the length of the obit.
If it is short, I wonder if anyone really loved them.
What did they look like and what was happening
at the precise moment when they died?

Still Life with Rose (script excerpt)
- Suzanne Costello & Stuart Pimsler

In this book's introduction, I mention my wonderment at John Graham-Pole's ability to stay uplifted while experiencing the loss of so many patients. As our work with oncology and hospice caregivers expanded, I continued to marvel at their resilience. We wanted to know more about these individuals who were working at the precipice of life and death. Why did they choose this work? How did they cope? During this same period, I was also searching for answers about my own recent losses. In 1990, a close friend and colleague, Ron "Aiji" Kajiwara, died of an AIDS-related illness. Ron, a design director for *Vogue* magazine, had been SPDT's scene designer in New York City and continued in that role when we moved to Columbus. The set designer for

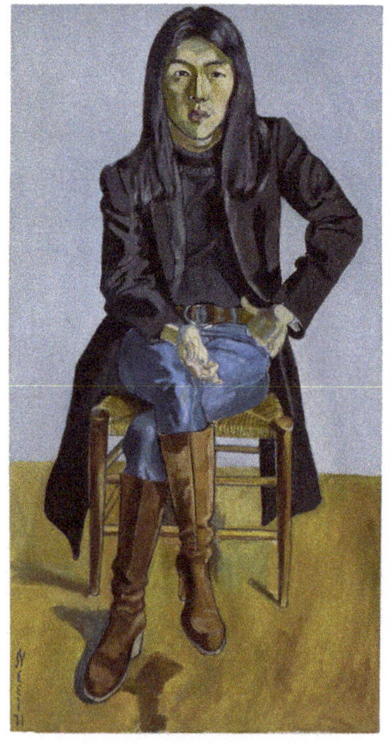

Ron Kajiwara (1971)
Reproduction of original painting
by artist Alice Neel

Swimming to Cecile and other works, Ron was also my design mentor and inspiration for viewing the world in new ways. His public modesty and introversion belied his ability and joy for creating sophisticated worlds in stunning monochromatic tonalities. During his last days, Ron told me he hoped to return as a rainbow. After his cremation, while walking on the beach in Provincetown, Massachusetts, I witnessed my first fogbow—sometimes called a white rainbow.

Soon after Ron's passing, my father died at Rosary Hill, a hospice founded in 1901 by Mother Mary Alphonsa Lathrop, aka Rose Hawthorne, daughter of American novelist Nathaniel Hawthorne. Unlike Ron, my father, Lenny, had decided to not challenge his illness—throat cancer—continuing to smoke after receiving a laryngectomy. His panache on the dance floor accompanied him in his final moments, which I experienced during our last visit. My father was in a morphine-induced slumber when Suzanne and I arrived at Rosary Hill. His stark room, featuring a large crucifix over his bed, was populated by the caring presence of Dominican nuns. When Lenny awoke, we were greeted with a generous "God be with you" delivered by a friar wearing a traditional robe and hood. After the friar's exit, I assured my groggy, wide-eyed father that he had not been sent to the wrong resting place—he was still here, still Jewish. I didn't realize that my propensity for dark-humored relief would find kinship throughout our future work with professional caregivers.

In 1996, with funding provided by the Academy of Medicine of Columbus, Ohio and the Franklin County Foundation, Suzanne and I presented a series of *Caring for the Caregiver* workshops throughout the metropolitan area. We had developed these workshops as our initial response to how we as artists could best serve the needs of caregivers. John Graham-Pole had opened the door, inviting us into the community, and since that moment, we continued to find creative outlets for the caregivers' emotional stresses. By exploring the power of touch, movement, and storytelling, they were finding new opportunities to refresh their practices while strengthening connections with their colleagues and patients. I have already discussed many of our *Caring for the Caregiver* exercises in Chapter 4.

In Columbus, we presented these workshops in coordination with three healthcare facilities: Hospice of Grant Riverside, Mt. Carmel

Hospice, and Kobacker House—a 32-bed inpatient hospice. The three hospices had staff at ten different facilities. Participants in the workshops included physicians, nurses, social workers, psychotherapists, hospice staff, hospice volunteers, medical students, nursing students, hospital chaplains, persons with life-threatening illnesses, and their families and friends.

At the conclusion, we invited participants from the ten workshops to join us in the creation of an original stage work. This would be our first attempt to create a new production with professional caregivers. The cast included 12 seasoned practitioners with ongoing responsibilities in the hospice community, including four nurses, two chaplains, two social workers, one doctor, one art therapist, one psychologist, and one hospice volunteer. One nurse had experienced our work previously during a three-thousand-member convening of the Oncology Nursing Society at the Cincinnati Convention Center; she was an enthusiastic advocate of the project.

At our first rehearsal, after introductions, the cast members talked about their professional challenges. The shortage of beds, insurance protocols, insufficient time with patients, and always giving support without receiving any were common themes. The one topic uniting all the participants was their deep connection to their patients/clients— those individuals who had left indelible impressions. Each caregiver expressed the sacred nature of sharing stories and moments with patients nearing death. The cast rejoiced in those vivid memories but struggled with their plentitude of loss. They were joined by a desire to grieve their beloved patients. How could they achieve this when community and personal mourning rituals were neither formalized nor encouraged?

This was a first moment for Suzanne and me to focus our work on a singular topic. Would we be able to find creative outlets for addressing the unresolved mourning of dedicated caregivers? We began with wanting to know more about each caregiver's daily routines, both at and away from the workplace. They talked about favorite herbal teas, walking the dog, baths by candlelight, and the private shedding of tears. One daily habit shared by most of the cast members was the reading of obituaries. Initially cultivated as a workplace necessity—

had someone died since their last shift?—many had become well-versed in the styles and content of how an individual's passing was publicly reported. We asked everyone to write about their particular interest in obituaries. Next, we invited the cast to imagine authoring their own obituaries.

> *I have a pretty short name, so I think I'll be able to have lots of space for lots of information. If I'm still living in the same apartment, I'll describe the different rooms and the great southern exposure. I would certainly mention my doctor's name and their care of me—as a review for the next patient. Oh, Dr. K. really knows how to look in your eyes as he is talking to you. And oh yes, my three dogs whom I love very much and could survive me.*

We shaped our new work, revising and editing the cast's writings and discussions. To protect and honor confidentiality, all references to their patients remained anonymous. The movement material, developed in collaboration with the performers, was a mixture of gestures and behaviors inspired by their workplaces. Multiple white sheets, a utilitarian workplace necessity, were integrated as an iconic symbol. A local dance writer commented:

> *Another moment that cuts to the bone involves sheets as props. Dancers lie down on top of a white sheet, a partner hovering above them invoking the myriad scenes in hospital beds across the country at this very moment. At once, the group jumps up and starts shaking out the sheets, laying them on the ground, violently ripping them back off the ground, and laying them down again and again. The fabric whips audibly and the metaphor is chilling. Each sheet represents a patient and a death.*[52]

The work's red costumes, its ending, and its eventual title were suggested by an honoring ritual from one of the hospices. After a patient's passing, the bedding is replaced with a clean white sheet topped with a red rose. Barring demand, the bed is left vacant for twenty-four hours. *Still Life with Rose* was premiered in Columbus, Ohio with other SPDT works in an evening poetically titled Simchas and Sorrows.[53]

Many of the *Still Life with Rose* cast—newly dubbed the "Red Dancers"—had never performed before. Their sheer joy and satisfaction were readily apparent. During post-performance talkbacks, colleagues and other audience members expressed their gratitude. The piece was a rare glimpse into the emotional duress of the working care-giver, while exposing their vulnerabilities. Suzanne and I were enthralled by the risks taken by the cast and proud that the work was so enthusiastically received. We invited the cast to accompany us on an upcoming national tour, sharing *Still Life with Rose* with new audiences in other U.S. locations.

On tour, as the Red Dancers grew more confident, the work became more impactful. The cast was grateful to have a safe place to share tender memories from their encounters with the dying. Communities continued to express their thanks for uncovering the caregivers' humanity and fragility. We felt compelled to expand our creative partnership with caregivers while continuing to challenge ourselves artistically. Emboldened by the success of *Still Life with Rose*, we started to imagine our next project.

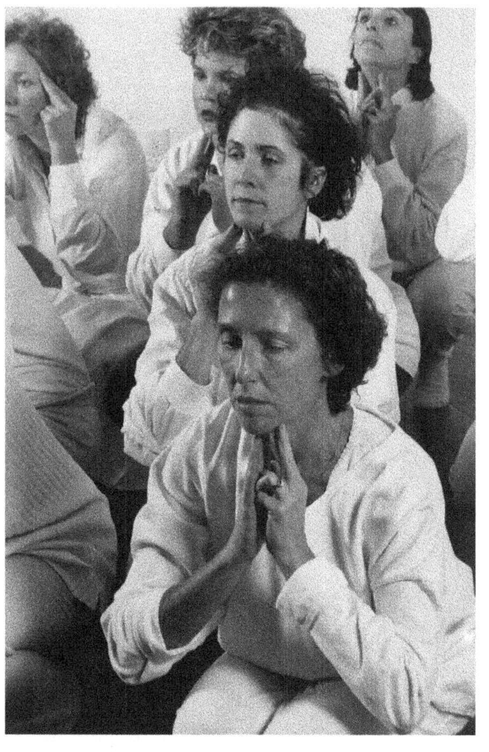

Still Life with Rose
Cast of Hospice Caregivers,
Columbus, Ohio
Photo Credit: Brad Feinknopf (1996)

CHAPTER SEVEN

Out of This World/
The Life After Life Project

Even in normal times, we survive on ironic,
dark humor because we deal with death and sickness...
But these days, the jokes are sometimes so sharp as to bite.[54]

- Thomas Kirsch

The COVID-19 pandemic confronted professional caregivers around the globe with unprecedented challenges. Caregivers were on the front lines trying to save lives as the world sought vaccines and treatments for combating the coronavirus. The *Journal of the American Medical Association* reported that of 138 patients studied at a Wuhan, China hospital, 29 percent were healthcare workers.[55] In the U.S., due to inconsistencies in tracking and testing, the infection rate among professional caregivers was first assessed through state coronavirus websites. Rates ranged from a low of five percent in Pennsylvania to as high as twenty percent in Ohio and New Hampshire.[56] An early report by the U.S. Centers for Disease Control found that over 9200 American professional caregivers had been infected.[57] The coronavirus has intensified the need for protecting and healing those who continue to care for others. Public and private sectors collaborated to address the undersupply of personal protective equipment—safety masks, gowns, and eye shields. Spiritual uplift resounded as neighborhoods offered public tributes and thanks to their local caregivers: an eight-foot-high THANK YOU on a fence near a Queens, New York, hospital; a mural thanking Dallas nurses; a six-ton sand sculpture of a healthcare worker cradling the world in New Jersey; cars honking their horns in thanks in Owasso, Oklahoma; fresh bouquets delivered daily at hospital entrances; and songs of gratitude echoing outside of healthcare facilities around the globe.

These days, being overwhelmed by a disease with no cure is a rare occurrence. However, the reality of life-threatening illness and lives lost is an ever-present condition for caregivers even during more "normal times." There are few institutional solutions for addressing the caregivers' long work hours, despair, and grief. Caregivers are superheroes in humble attire. Their workplaces are inundated with life-saving tasks and little time for reflection. Sometimes the mere reminder to take a deep breath feels luxurious and reminiscing about a recent patient an indulgence. But when Suzanne and I have facilitated reflective discussions about patients, caregivers have spoken eloquently, grateful for this healing opportunity.

Caregivers often espouse personal rituals while witnessing a patient's death. Some whisper, "It's OK to go, you can go, go, go." Another looks up and thinks, "Bon voyage." And a hospice nurse gently hums at the moment of a patient's demise. Caregivers rejoice in hopes of less suffering for patients even after their demise—a wish for peace, *after*.

Following the notion of "after," we began to imagine a new performance work on the heels of *Still Life with Rose*. Our initial musings led us to consider the mystery of continuity after death. We familiarized ourselves with a diversity of religious and philosophical writings addressing the afterlife. There is unanimity on the one hand—everyone dies—and discord on the other—what lies beyond? What happens after life? Does dying transport us to another location?

* * * * *

Bart Ehrman, Professor of Religious Studies at the University of North Carolina, was interviewed last year to discuss his new book—*Heaven and Hell: A History of the Afterlife*. While unmasking the traditional notions of codified afterlifes—Greek, Jewish or Christian—Ehrman highlights some selected personal visions. He is drawn to the trial of Socrates and his conversations with colleagues as he awaited his death sentence. For Socrates, death was one of two possibilities. A continuation of living—somewhere—and spending time with familiar individuals who have also died. Ehrman imagined Socrates enjoying the unexpected opportunities to converse with Homer and other Greek luminaries. However, an alternate possibility would be a deep, dreamless sleep. Either way, Socrates was confident that everything would be just fine after an individual's demise. And Ehrman in 2020, believed exactly the same thing.[58]

Extensive Gallup polling about the afterlife began in the 1980s and since that time Americans have remained steadfast in their outlooks. Nearly eighty percent of individuals polled believe in some form of afterlife.[59] The mysteries shrouding these beliefs focus on desires to know—Do the dead remain dead? Where do they go? Can they return? Reincarnation, resurrection, rebirth, immortality, and the inexplicable pervade our thinking. Early Judaic doctrines describe the specific afterlife task required to reach a central meeting place:

> Even to this day, it is a custom in the Diaspora to bury a person with a small stick, or dowel, placed in the casket. Since the operating belief is that the resurrection will take place in the Holy Land, at the designated time of redemption, the person will be able to burrow through the earth to the Land of Israel and participate fully in the miracle of resurrection.[60]

The Tewa, a group of Pueblo Native Americans, describe another after-dying ritual. It starts with senior relatives of the same sex dressing the corpse in traditional clothing.

> Moccasins are reversed, and a bit of food, whatever they most enjoyed eating in life, is wrapped in cotton and placed in their left armpit. These two acts are done because everything in the afterworld— the world beneath this one—is reversed. The amount of food will vary with the individual; if he has been highly regarded in life, only a small amount is placed in the armpit, for the road to the afterworld will be straight.[61]

Musings on afterlife were intriguing, and in some instances provided relief from the subject's austerity. Author Thomas Lynch, lifelong director of a Michigan funeral parlor, has much to say about the business of dying. In his book, *The Undertaking: Life Studies from the Dismal Trade*, he opines about death, mourning—"mourning is a romance in reverse"—and afterlife.[62] Lynch has a deep respect for death and his literary sensibility dares to embrace dying's beauty, humor, and inevitability. In one darkly humorous passage, Lynch suggests the possibility of recycling cremains into some tangible memorabilia—"cremorialization." He elaborates through such examples as recycling the ashes of a fisherman into a sinker or hook, ashes of a gambler becoming dice and playing chips, car buffs turned into gearshift knobs, and for the more mundane, a pair of bookends.

While processing much research about life's aftermath, we remained committed to a creative filter that would provide some pragmatic salve for caregiver participants. We reframed our inquiries in response to the caregivers' workplace, asking: Are there personal coping mechanisms following a loss? Do professional caregivers live their lives differently once a patient has died? How do memories of patients live on for caregivers—in their bodies, in their voices? Our approach to this new project, *Out of This World/The Life After Life Project (OOTW)*, developed by exploring "the life the living live after the patient has died."[63]

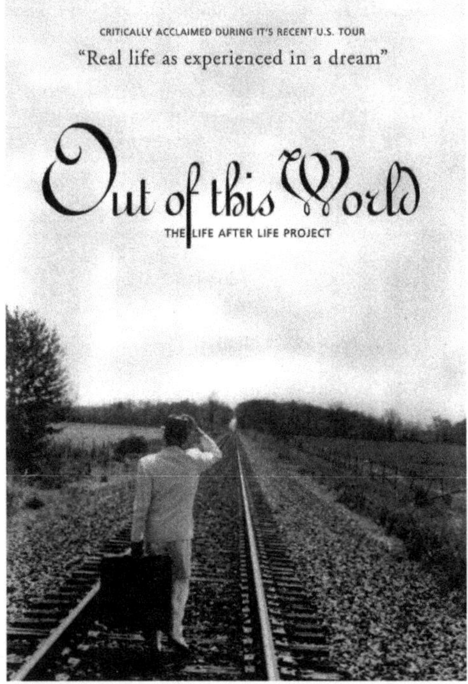

OUT OF THIS WORLD/
The Life After Life Project
(1998-2001) Poster/Flyer
Graphic design: Michael Howett

The University of Arizona, with major funding from the Lila Wallace Reader's Digest Arts Partners Fund, commissioned *Out of This World/ The Life After Life Project*. After its 1998 premiere in Tucson, the piece toured to Pittsburgh, Pennsylvania; Gainesville, Florida; Columbus, Ohio; and Minneapolis, Minnesota. In each city, we invited local caregivers and artists to join our core artistic team, which included composer Ingram Marshall, filmmaker Al Laus, lighting designer Patricia Mahoney, vocalists Madeline Rivera and Ajamu Mutima, and scenic designer Joe McGrath. We recruited participants by presenting *Caring for the Caregiver* workshops at hospices, hospitals, and other healthcare venues in every host community. By the time *OOTW* had its final performance in 2001, we had worked with nearly four hundred caregivers and artists in the five partnering cities.

Our starting point for every rendition of *OOTW* asked participants to invite a deceased patient, family member, or friend to join them. For many of the caregivers, this was a formidable task. Many had helped thousands of patients close their eyes for the last time throughout their careers. We urged them to consider one patient who lived on through valued advice, a singular phrase, a cherished expression, a posture, a gesture, or a specific song that could be recalled and expressed. We invited participants to share their deceased partners with the rest of the cast. The process resounded in grief, longing, and tributes—an opportunity to imagine immortality as a memory.

The following is an excerpt from the script for the Columbus version of *OOTW*. We asked each performer to write about an imagined meeting with their deceased partner—recalling an activity or conversation that began with the words, "I dreamed I saw…" By editing the individual scenarios into a group text, we created a community poem of memories.

    Lindy
She touched my shoulder

    Enas
And I said, "Let me tell everyone you're here!"

    Lisa
She was cooking.

    All
Of course!

    Lisa
And the grandkids were playing and being loud.

    All
Of course!

Lisa
And I was watching.

Clare
We told stories about what we had missed.

Nat
We learned that I was completing your journey.

Susan
She said....

Lisa
Come on you guys, come and eat.

All
Of course!

Clare
She said, "I know you will succeed."

Diane
He said, "You are so special."

Liz
She said we could talk, and I could hear her voice.

Beth
He said, "Never lease, you lose too much money."

Nat
She said, "Learn to forgive and enjoy."

Enas
Then she said her time was up.

Susan
I wished

Diane
We had more days like this.

Lisa
I wished I didn't feel like such a stranger.

Nat
I wished she had been strong enough to love me this way while
she was alive.

> Beth
> I wished I had more time with him.

> Clare
> I wished it was real.

> Susan
> As the dream was ending

> Beth
> A waiter came out of nowhere and told my dad it was time to leave.

> Nat
> We were humming a lullaby.

> Diane
> He held me.

> Lindy
> She whispered in my ear.

> Liz
> We smiled to ourselves.

> Enas
> She left.

> Lisa
> Everything dissolved.

> Clare
> And I went home alone.

A participating Presbyterian minister described *OOTW's* creative process as being similar to her own work. "My job is to listen to their relatives and then to tell their story. To make the death public. To let others look through a window and see them asleep and to feel their ultimate stillness."[64] Other participants spoke of having their memories jogged, surprised by a certain moment during a rehearsal. A Minneapolis nurse had lost her mother at the age of three. Moving to a specific music selection in *OOTW* triggered her memory of a childhood music box. "It's like the memory was in my body. I don't remember how my mother looked or smelled or how she talked. But her being is in me and I didn't even know it."[65]

While the five renditions of *OOTW* reflected each city's unique cast, there were certain repeating artistic elements. Mark Strand, a Pulitzer Prize-winning American author and the nation's fourth poet laureate, granted us permission to integrate his poem "Farewell" as text for the music composed by Ingram Marshall. The poem's three sections inform the structural spine for *OOTW* while suggesting theme variations and tonalities. Vocalist Madeline Rivera, perched on a swing high above the stage, sings Strand's opening lines.

> It is true, as someone has said, that in
> A world without Heaven all is farewell.
> Whether you wave your hand or not,
> It is farewell, and if no tears come to your eyes
> It is still farewell, and if you pretend not to notice,
> Hating what passes, it is still farewell.
> Farewell no matter what. And the palms as they lean
> Over the green, bright lagoon, and the pelicans
> Diving, and the glistening bodies of bathers resting
> Are stages in an ultimate stillness.[66]

Another constant was a black and white film staged on railroad tracks in a rural location near Columbus, Ohio. The film, created for *OOTW*, afforded a dreamlike metaphor for the work's subject matter, described below in my journal excerpt. The *OOTW* film cast included the professional caregivers from *Still Life with Rose*, our daughter Sophia Cecile Pimsler, vocalist Madeline Rivera, Suzanne, and myself. Without acquiring a formal permit, we persuaded a local farmer to let us use a portion of his land where the railroad tracks passed through. For a variety of reasons, including the fact that we were trespassing through interstate commerce, wary of local deer hunters, and had chosen to wear summer-like costumes, we were motivated to film as quickly as possible. During two wintry November days we shot the film, avoiding passing trains while benefiting from a brief snow shower—perfect ambience for the film's ethereal imagery.

Upon completing the film shoot, I reflected on the day. The repeating motif for the short film was a man dressed in white, walking on railroad tracks.

Driving home, I had a little taste of out-of-body-ness that surely comes from being encapsulated in an intense, solitary location for an extended period. I can't let go of the walk. Walking with a suitcase on railroad tracks, walking away from the camera, my back exposed—over and over again. My caregiver friends, the guides, dressed in white, standing nearby watching me walk. I never look at them. I am unattended but determined. Walking toward somewhere that I never get to, that I had never been to, and I could only speculate what might be waiting. A last respite, a brief dance and turn with my daughter on the tracks before continuing on my walk toward a disappearing perspective.[67]

The Minneapolis version of *OOTW* included a narrator (Maria Cheng) who added a new dimension to the group of guides. Maria's closing text was spoken to another younger guide, nine-year-old Sophia Pimsler. The dialogue references some of Mark Strand's poem while recalling images from the opening film.

MARIA. Hello…Goodbye…Farewell…Adieu…Here…There Go in any direction and you will return to the main drag. I don't know about you, but I'm dying for a parade, even if no one is there. I will see their outlines as I pass through the outskirts. Carrying one very, very tiny invisible suitcase filled with fragments of before. The end will look like…I dare you to tell me. Everyone dies differently.

SOPHIA. That's the beauty of it.

MARIA. From far away, life looked to be simpler back in the town you started from. Look, there in the window are mom and dad.

Our contribution to afterlife ideology was realized through the stories of caregivers and individuals. Their memories of deceased individuals who lived on shaped their stories. Mary Hamaan-Roland, the mayor of Apple Valley, a nearby Minnesota city, who attended *OOTW's* last performance on January 26, 2001, wrote to us: "The democracy on stage was poignant and inspiring due to the incredible diversity of cultural belief systems expressed through the performance."

CHAPTER EIGHT

WASH: Working with Artists, Sharing the Healing

*We can't begin to approach whole-person needs without
going back a step and dealing with the care of the caregivers.
Through their own healing, caregivers come to understand
that patients can heal whether they are recovering or dying.*

- Sandy Heywood, Tucson psychologist and cast member,
Out of This World/ The Life After Life Project.

In the aftermath of *Out of This World's* last performance, Suzanne and I reflected on our ten-year history of working in arts and medicine. It had been a wide-eyed journey through a community and workplace perpetually in emotional strife. Outlets offering relief and rejuvenation were scarce. Our work with caregivers had taught us much about a field we had only previously experienced as consumers. Caregivers were often exhausted, on the brink of leaving their professions—the result of grueling training and dire work conditions. There were minimal institutional protocols for dealing with the emotionally fraught issues that impacted them. The workplace culture, beginning with their educational challenges (discussed in Chapter 2), discouraged public admissions about sadness, regret, and failure. Caregivers were expected to tough it out and seek solace behind the scenes.

With these insights, it was no surprise that our work was received with such grand enthusiasm and relief. The more work we took on, the more requests we received. We realized that there was an inordinate demand for supporting the wellness of caregivers—and with that demand, an opportunity for more artists to become involved. We became interested in expanding our work by sharing our knowledge and techniques with other artists. Our tenure in arts and medicine/health had grown through a series of trusted partnerships and community collaborations. These prior relationships informed a desire to be mindful of how to expand our sphere of influence. Working with healthcare providers was part of a larger arts discipline—community-based art making—that entailed different presumptions about process and outcomes.

In shaping our next endeavor, we adhered to two community-based principles while reaching out to interested artists. The traditional model of a singular artistic vision presented to the masses was not appropriate. Working in the community of caregivers necessitated a willingness to shift the model and embrace a first precept of a community-based practice—from artist for the people to artist of the people. Participating artists had to be disposed to listen to their potential collaborators and facilitate creative expression in concert with them. This dynamic shift required a pivot from the artist as an individual deliverer to acting as a facilitator and organizer. In the realm of community-based art making, public participation and artistic creation are mutually interdependent. The process joins aesthetic considerations with other community outcomes in gauging success. The awareness, emotional relief, and resolve for change that a caregiver may discover through a creative process are as significant as a finished piece of art.[68]

This first principle impelled creative expression to emerge from the lives of all participants rather than from the vision of the professional artist. Logically, the second principle demanded that caregivers, as community participants, needed to be more than spectators.[69] Working with caregivers required an altered collaborative paradigm. Artists shouldn't be the ones speaking on behalf of their caregiver-partners. Professional caregivers have the capacity to explore their own creative lives and to resound in their own creative expression. We would challenge caregivers to be active participants, rather than observers, in a creative process expressing issues from their workplaces.

It became apparent that adhering to the two community-based guidelines, as well as our prior experiences with professional caregivers, required a format where artists would learn in partnership with caregivers. It would be presumptuous to imagine that artists could know the workplace concerns of caregivers. *WASH: Working with Artists, Sharing the Healing* introduced both caregivers and artists to the dynamic of collaboration across their respective disciplines. Artists were expected to share their techniques for making art while caregivers related their workplace experiences.

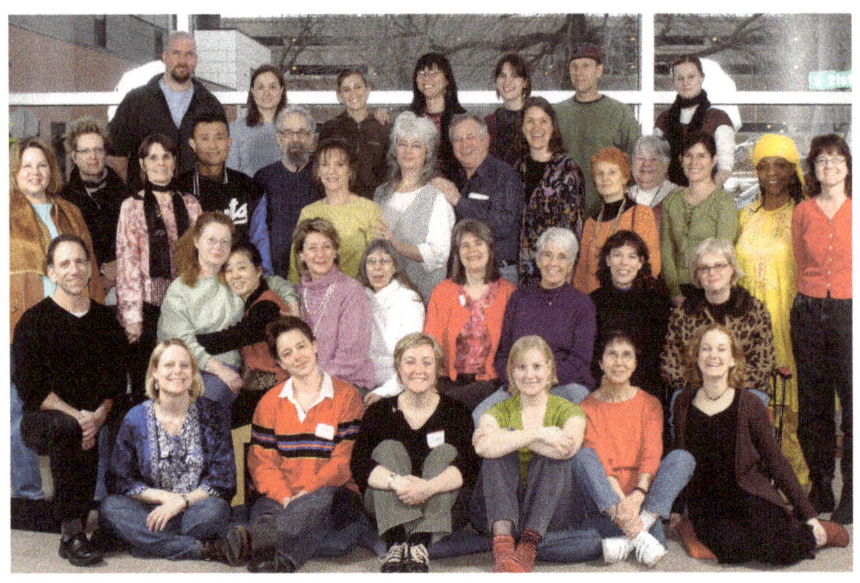

WASH Alumni—Artists and Professional Caregivers
Photo Credit: Howard Bell (2003)

WASH premiered March 15, 2002, unfolding over a three-day period with 16½ hours of instruction. The National Endowment for the Arts supported *WASH* during its six-year history. We selected equal numbers of caregivers and artists, anticipating that duet collaborations might offer the most robust engagements. We invited participants to apply for admission by submitting responses describing their work and aspirations for enrolling. We wanted to know why artists were interested in working with caregivers, and similarly, why caregivers wanted to explore creative expression. Caregivers paid a registration fee for the 3-day program. For artists, we asked that in lieu of the fee they use their work as currency by providing 1-2 in-service programs after the conclusion of the workshop. These programs were presented in collaboration with a caregiver partner from *WASH*. Each duo was expected to report on their inservice/art projects during the next 12 months.

Throughout our projects with caregivers, we had learned that having a community advocate-partner was critical—an organization, institution, or individual implanted in the healthcare field who supported our vision. Fortunately, as we planned *WASH*, we worked in consort with Marge Maddux, former director of dance at the University of

Minnesota, and Howard Bell, retired executive director of Pathways. (A Minneapolis-based resource center, Pathways offers complementary therapies, emotional support and other educational resources for persons living with life-threatening illnesses).

During our tenure at UM as adjunct faculty members, Marge supported us in our work as university instructors and as community-engaged artists. Howard and Pathways had previously commissioned SPDT for other projects including *Moving Inquiries*, a site-specific performance at the Weisman Art Museum.[70] In 2007, Howard again commissioned SPDT to create a new work, *Undercovers*.

During its tenure, *WASH* facilitated and mentored the work of nearly 200 caregivers and artists. Participating artists were broadly represented across disciplinary interests, including writers, poets, book illustrators, dancers, choreographers, sculptors, painters, musicians, vocalists, visual artists, actors, and directors. Caregivers were also diversely represented; we engaged doctors, nurses, students, social workers, psychotherapists, counselors, pastors, and hospice massage and respiratory therapists.

In shaping the format for *WASH*, Suzanne and I believed that maximizing experiential time was critical. We wanted to augment hands-on, collaborative experience between artists and caregivers. Our goal was to expose attending caregivers to the unique creative processes of the participating artists. Similarly, we hoped that the artists would learn about the varying workplace concerns of the caregivers. To optimize attendees' collaborative time, we directed the three-day event with a very light hand—attempting to ignite possibilities, then get out of the way.

As with all of our projects, *WASH* began with participant introductions. Artists were asked to describe their work and share examples of their medium. Caregivers spoke about their workplaces and the patients they cared for. We asked all participants to address their reasons for coming to *WASH* and what they hoped to learn. A group movement exercise, intended as both an icebreaker and as a non-verbal opportunity for saying "Hello," followed these introductions. The group then transitioned from moving together into their first creative exchanges.

In forming teams for these first collaborations, we directed individuals into quartets comprising two caregivers and two artists. We asked each group to reintroduce themselves. Caregivers were asked to articulate one unresolved workplace issue that they spend time thinking about. Artists listened and then suggested creative responses for addressing the caregivers' concerns. Next, we provided open-studio work time for each group to collaborate. The outcomes of the collaborations were presented to the group, either as live performance/demonstrations or as verbal summaries. Short warmup movement exercises interspersed with differently populated creative-exchange groups continued as the basic format throughout *WASH*. Guest speakers from complementary, alternative, and integrative arts and healing programs were also invited to present their work.

In planning *WASH*, Suzanne and I felt strongly about the need to address the nitty gritty of how to get a foot in the door of a healthcare venue. While the traditions and protocols of western medicine were shifting, the bureaucracy of healthcare delivery remained steadfast. We had learned much about:

- Identifying the decision-makers at healthcare venues

- Crafting a proposal

- The requirements of Continuing Education Units—CEUs

- When and where to schedule an event

- Evaluations

- Requesting payment

- Building relationships

We knew that possessing brilliant creative ideas would not guarantee success for artists hoping to work in the field of arts and health. Understanding how to position their work in the healthcare marketplace and learning the business realities of that community were essential.

At the conclusion of *WASH*, each artist/caregiver partnership committed to presenting one creative program at the caregiver's site. Periodic progress reports were requested so that Suzanne and I could monitor activities while providing any necessary troubleshooting.

The successes of *WASH* were many—some individual and some institutional. For example, one musician started playing music at the bedside of her partner-caregiver's patients. This eventually led to the musician being hired to play music in the hospital's surgical unit. Another counselor reported integrating drawing into her individual healing practice and using story circles in group settings.

A hospice nurse working with a visual artist was deeply impacted. "I have a new job—halftime with hospice and halftime with the Foundation working on projects that bring together healing and the arts. What I learned most from the weekend is to be quiet, and listen, and allow people to just experience. I'm very frustrated with people thinking that artists interested in working at hospice could volunteer their time. I had a conversation with our medical director in which he suggested that perhaps artists interested in working at hospice could volunteer. I asked him, "What if we asked you to volunteer your time as the medical director?" He laughed but he was forced to reflect on it.

The well-meaning medical director, his colleagues, and other caregivers continue to recognize the importance of the arts in health. Dissatisfaction with the delivery and outcomes of western medicine has influenced the public's desire for a more integrated approach to health. Creative expression is being prescribed to provide comfort, relief, and wellness in partnership with evidence-based medicine. The holistic pursuit of body, mind, and spirit, undertaken by dancers and other seekers of creative expression, is now being recognized and valued in many parts of the medical community.

In 2007, the Society for the Arts in Healthcare (SAH)[71] partnered with the Joint Commission (www.jointcommission.org: the national accreditation agency for healthcare) and Americans for the Arts (www.americansforthearts.org: a national arts advocacy agency) to conduct a survey regarding arts programs in U.S. healthcare facilities. Of the 1807 institutions responding, nearly 50 percent reported having ongoing arts programs in their facilities.[72] These programs vary across a range of categories that include training and education for professional caregivers, caring for personal caregivers, art at patients' bedsides and in public spaces, performing arts created with caregivers, art therapies, and environmental aesthetics.[73]

CHAPTER NINE

Learning

*I believe the arts are a service industry. We doctor different things.
We doctor the invisible hurt. We mend the phantom pain.
I believe we are essential for humanity.*[74]

- Jonathan Majors (Actor)

Suzanne and I continue to create pathways to communities that once seemed very far away, or for us uncharted. With every new project, we spend much time researching the populations with which we'll collaborate. Each community of caregivers is unique, influenced by the particular challenges of those they care for. I know now that research will never fully prepare me. Nothing can substitute for the ability to see, hear, and experience live participants in a space—sitting in the magic circle.

In 2012, a nurse manager from North Memorial Hospital's newly established Stroke Center contacted us. She had participated in our workshop at the annual conference of the Oncological Nursing Society. This same individual, a long-tenured oncology nurse, had suffered a stroke in the ensuing years. She asked us to work with stroke survivors and their caregivers, many of whom were life partners. It was to be our first endeavor with this population.

From an early age, I remembered my grandmother's stroke and how her mouth seemed to sag on one side in the aftermath. At the time, I vaguely understood the reasons given for her inability to articulate words and complete full sentences. The afterimage of her slumped in a chair with a dislocated gaze accompanied me into the project.

I also read about the physical conditions caused by a stroke. The range of disabilities was vast, from partial paralysis to death. Hippocrates was the first healer to observe strokes. During his time, stroke was called apoplexy, which in Greek means "struck down by violence."

It wasn't until the 20th century that the cause of strokes was linked most often to a lack of blood supply to the brain—cerebral vascular accident (CVA) or "brain attack."[75]

How would we work with a population that might have severe physical and cognitive limitations? On the day before our first workshop, my nervous, anticipatory energy led me to the dictionary. I remain enthralled by words, even after a 40-year career as a dancer persistently mining the non-verbal. The Merriam Webster Dictionary has 12 definitions for stroke used as a noun and more for its usage as a verb. They include an array of movement actions, from "a propelling movement" (the stroke of an oar) to "an act of caressing" to "a heartbeat." Instead of settling for physical limitations, I hoped to find ways, even limited ones, to explore movement with the stroke survivors and their caregivers. Suzanne suggested we title our new program with stroke survivors, *Meaning in Movement.*

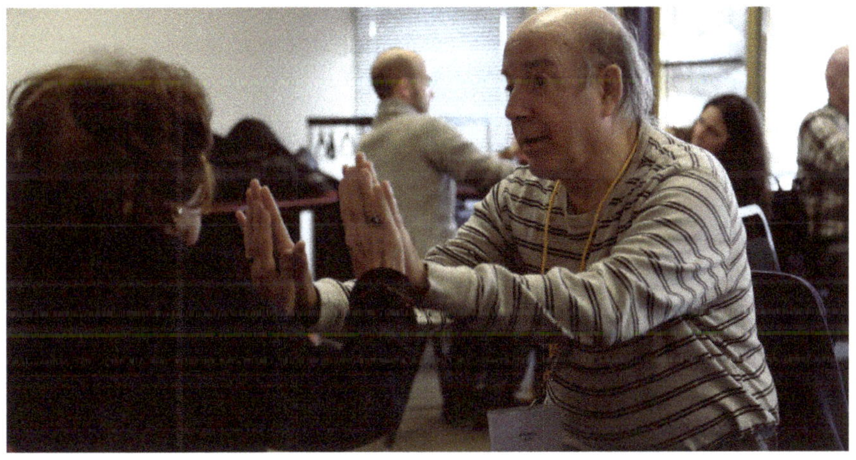

Meaning in Movement workshop, Alzheimer's Association,
Louisville, Kentucky
Photo Credit: Stuart Pimsler (2016)

During our month-long workshop with the stroke population, we observed, respected, and followed the lead set by the group. Each pair of participants had their own limitations depending on their existing physical and mental disabilities. Some struggled with verbal articulation, some had lost mobility of a limb, and a few relied on wheelchairs. The common denominator for each duet was the noticeable degree of outward support shown by the able caregiver (often a life partner) and the loving bonds that seemed to exist. Our first instinct was to facilitate physical activities that allowed the able individuals to lead their stroke partners. Participants were surprised and energized by the challenge to move in unfamiliar ways, if only minimally.

In one workshop session, we asked the stroke survivors to close their eyes. We hoped to facilitate an exercise that would require the able individual to lead his or her stroke survivor on an eyes-shut movement journey. The group voiced concern over our directions as many stroke survivors struggle with maintaining balance. In the moment, we switched leadership roles, asking the stroke survivors to lead their more able partner. It was a revelation for us and a turning point for the group. After months and years of sustaining a predictable caregiver-patient relationship, we had altered the dynamic. It empowered the stroke survivor to make sense of where they were in their bodies and fulfill a task. Their movements, even with severe limitations, were being recognized and infused with a goal—guide your partner and move through the space. Everyone succeeded and appeared grateful for participating in roles lost since experiencing their strokes.

* * * * *

In the United States and across the globe, arts-in-medicine programs are attracting interest and new respect. The opportunity to present our work internationally has broadened our learning insights about healthcare delivery in other countries. These cross-cultural collaborations have affirmed how the process of artmaking resounds universally in meaning and appreciation. We have presented our *Caring for the Caregiver* workshops in Canada, Israel, Russia, and most recently, Mexico City.

In 2013, with support from the American Embassy in Mexico City, Roberto Cantoral Cultural Center, and the National Autonomous University of Mexico City (the largest university in Latin America), we presented our arts-in-medicine work at Hospital Infantil (Children's Hospital) de Mexico Federico Gomez and General Xoco Hospital. At the Hospital Infantil, our hosts, the director of nursing and a lead administrator, graciously bypassed our handshake offerings with generous embraces. Historic murals by Diego Rivera and other fabled Mexican artists were on display as we toured the hospital. Our hosts mentioned Mexico's tradition of public art, including Rivera's *History of Medicine in Mexico: The People's Demand for Better Health*. This 24' x 35' work, commissioned in 1951 to celebrate socialized healthcare, appears in the main lobby of another Mexico City healthcare venue, Hospital de la Raza.[76]

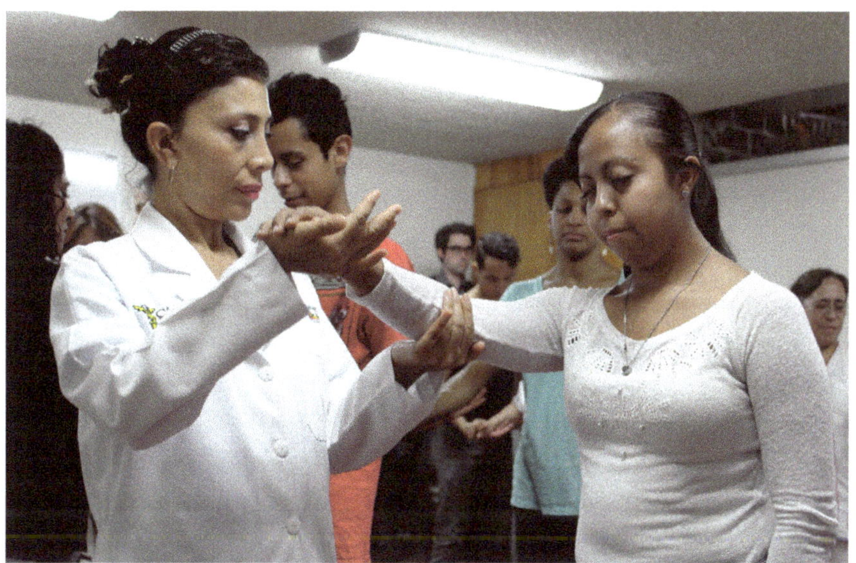

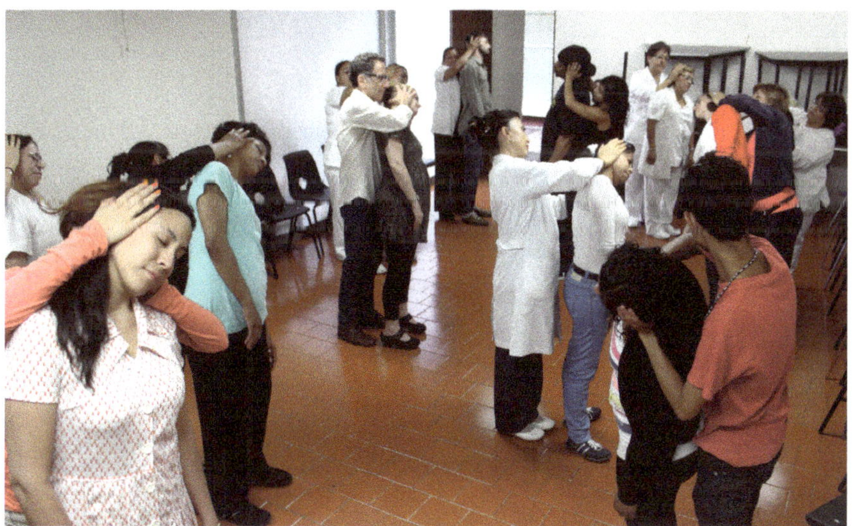

Caring for the Caregiver workshop, Xoco Hospital, Mexico City, Mexico
Photo Credit: Kari Mosel (2013)

105

We also learned of the "ninos del sismo" or the "children of the earthquake" legend, an inspiring story of survival after Mexico City's 1985 earthquake. Hospital Infantil had been the recovery site for 16 newborn infants rescued from earthquake rubble that claimed the lives of over 10,000 individuals. While the disaster killed many of their parents, the infants miraculously survived for up to one week under piles of debris. Hospital Infantil staff nurtured the surviving infants, becoming guardians of their wellbeing through adulthood.

At Xoco Hospital, we became further acquainted with Mexico's public health system. It was early morning, and a lengthy line of individuals was waiting outside the hospital's security gate. Everyone would receive medical care—eventually. Free healthcare for all Mexican citizens is a constitutional mandate. The hospital's director, a practicing physician, and the director of nursing escorted us through the security maze. Rather than murals, fading paint and aged signage adorned the Xoco Hospital walls. Patient rooms were stark, with antiquated, narrow iron beds positioned near each other. The beds' thin mattresses showed graphic indents from the bedspring coils. Patients, from children to seniors, were awaiting treatment as they enjoyed a modest lunch of hard-shelled tacos on paper plates.

Before making our way to the hospital's top floor, our hosts cautioned us to be ultra alert. Armed, uniformed soldiers guarded many of the rooms. Under Mexico's healthcare system, prisoners could receive free treatment, sometimes in the same venue as other citizens. This ward had been the site of a recent incident. A soldier had been cleaning his rifle and accidentally discharged it, hitting a nurse in her thigh. This particular caregiver stress was a first for us.

Even with the public demands of an overstressed system and outdated equipment, the caregivers in our workshops exuded generosity of spirit and compassion. I taxed my high school Spanish lessons beyond recognition, but the Mexican caregivers maintained a sense of humor, curiosity, and engagement. We moved together as they shared patient stories that resonated with familiarity regardless of locale.

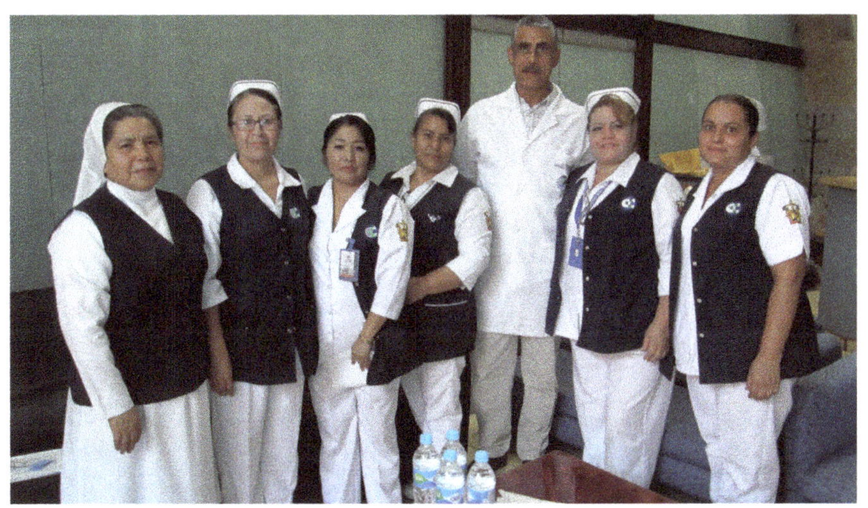

Caring for the Caregiver workshop, Guadalajara, Mexico
Photo Credit: Stuart Pimsler (2014)

Back in the United States, Suzanne was commissioned by Gilda's Club Twin Cities (a national cancer support community founded by *Saturday Night Live* comedian Gilda Radner, and her husband Gene Wilder) to create an original work, *LISTEN/Stories of Cancer* told through Movement, Music & Voice. Beginning in June of 2016, Suzanne facilitated a series of listening sessions at Gilda's Club, to learn about each person's experience with cancer. Participants included caregivers, family members and individuals dealing with different stages and types of cancer. From these initial stories, themes emerged that would eventually find their way into a new performance work. Participants spoke about cancer's impact on their lives. They also addressed their sense of isolation, exhaustion, and change of identity. One participant, interviewed at the conclusion of the project, said, "It offered an opportunity to reconnect me, as a breast cancer survivor, with my body that I had left sitting in the corner—to survive losing my image as a woman."

After the listening sessions, Suzanne directed a cast of 22 Gilda's Club participants and ten performing artists from Stuart Pimsler Dance & Theater. The final evening-length work was a powerful rendering of human courage and strength amid a life-threatening illness. A nurse practitioner in the cast had recently been diagnosed with metastatic breast cancer. She was particularly interested in participating in the project because her adolescent daughter was a dancer and she thought it would be a growth experience for both of them. The *LISTEN* Project was performed to sold-out audiences. Twin Cities Public Television documented Suzanne's process and created a 26-minute documentary—*LISTEN/Stories of Cancer and Resilience*. This public television special aired in February 2018 and was nominated for an Upper Midwest Emmy.[77]

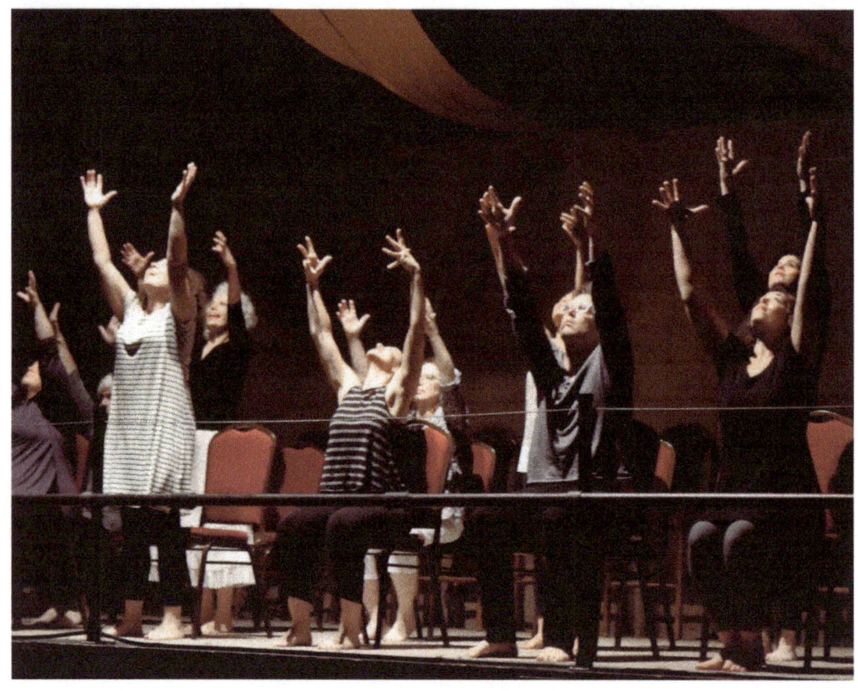

LISTEN/Stories of Cancer told through movement, music & voice
Photo Credit: V. Paul Virtucio (2016)

CHAPTER TEN

Foretell

What we miss—what we lose and what we mourn—
isn't it this that makes us who, deep down, we truly are?[78]

\- Sigrid Nunez, *The Friend*

The kindness of strangers can make a difference when touring the world. During a three-week residency in Kaoshiung, Taiwan, I worked with a selfless translator who had studied modern dance in the U.S. Before each class, the translator patiently coached my delivery of a new Mandarin phrase. As I facilitated daily movement warmups for my students, I would pepper directions with botched samplings of the native language. My students took great pleasure in listening to my heartfelt attempts and mispronunciations.

During a weekend recess, the translator invited me to lunch with her mother. Taiwanese cuisine is healthful and delicious, so I was surprised by the first offering—chou doufu (aka stinky tofu). As suggested by its title, stinky tofu is beyond subtle with a taste consistent with its aroma. I was relieved after my hosts assured me that the dish was intended more as a cultural experience—consumption was optional. Through our translator, I told the mother that stinky tofu reminded me of a family favorite—fried chicken livers with onions. Neither mother nor daughter inquired about the recipe.

By the end of our meal, I had learned about my hosts' family history, including their escape from the mainland. Arriving in Kaoshiung, the mother pursued studies to become a Taoist priestess. One of her skills was the reading of palms. The translator informed me that her mother hoped to read my palm. While still somewhat cautious from the stinky tofu encounter, I extended my palm toward the priestess. In silence, the three of us studied my hand, its hair thin lines like a roadmap to places unknown. The priestess zoomed in, tracing specific pathways with her index fingers. She asked her daughter for my permission to share her discoveries.

"Were you ever very ill as a child?" asked Priestess Mother.

"I had a bad case of scarlet fever and chicken pox with impetigo.

My measles were ordinary and some early heartburns were

caused by the previously referenced fried chicken livers," I responded.

"Did you ever come close to dying?" asked Priestess Mother.

"No," I said.

"You were supposed to," said Priestess Mother

I stared into my empty cup of tea for what seemed to be a very long time.

"You were supposed to die. But someone…a person very close to

you died so you could live," said Priestess Mother.

* * * * *

I had many dreams about my mother disappearing, becoming lost, or being injured during the year before her demise. For a time, I felt guilty about not warning her or trying to prevent her from crashing through the windshield. Did I really know my mother was going to die? My zayde could not accept the Judaic notion of *beshert*—divine providence mandating an event's inevitability. How did the Taoist priestess intuit this life-changing experience from my childhood? While aspiring to the secular realm of Judaism, the practice of religion has not been a part of my life since the loss of my mother. However, I have sought to embrace the magical, mystical and spiritual powers of creativity. The making of art has allowed me to experience, time and time again, how the unconscious can intuit what lies ahead. I no longer believe that forty-plus years of serendipitous juxtapositions can be merely explained as coincidences. The body sometimes knows before words are spoken.

Two years before launching our arts in health work, I created a new duet—*The Men from the Boys*. This work, a commentary on male power dynamics, includes a mock-heroic scene of prolonged dying. Inspired by old westerns and opera's extended scenes of deaths through song, my male counterpart and I die repeatedly as we cry out for our beloved. In the end, my enraged partner prevails, snapping my neck as the lights fade. While the tone of *The Men from the Boys* is quite different from *Swimming to Cecile*, each of these works is fascinated with the mysteries of death and dying. Did I know then that I would soon be immersed in a world where loss teases the caregiver's everyday experience?

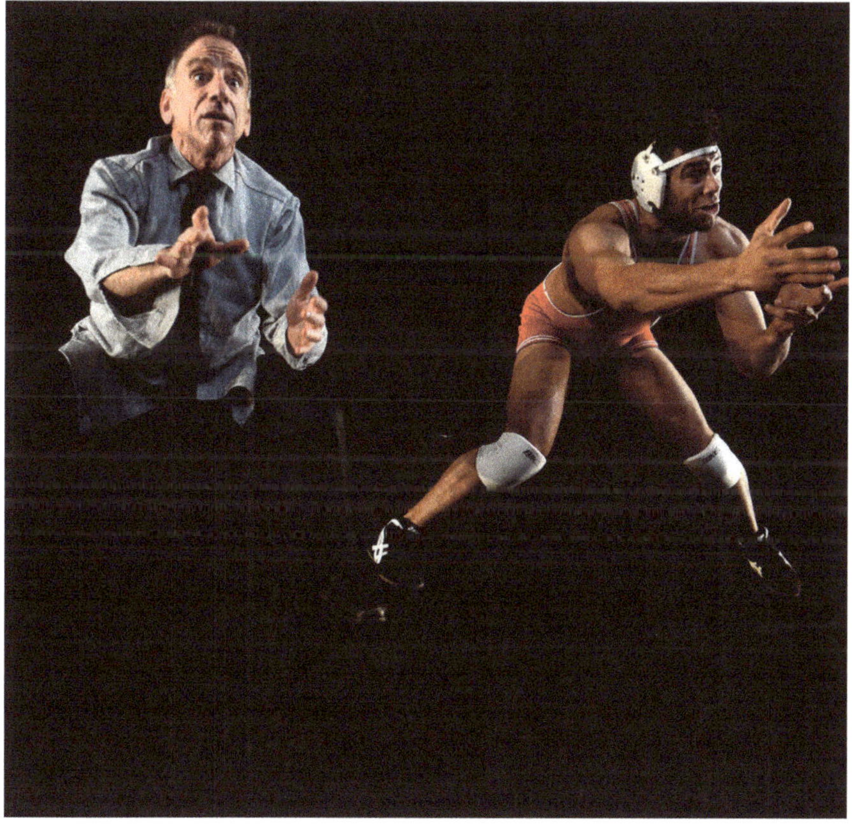

The Men from the Boys
Photo Credit: V. Paul Virtucio (2014)

Every day, my creative practice affords me the luxury and privilege of learning. In pursuit of new ideas, my job as an artist asks me to stay open, combining sensory awareness with intellectual curiosity. Artists are proficient problem solvers, embracing paradoxical situations. How do we discover movement possibilities for stroke survivors? Sometimes, this intersection of body and mind reverberates in questions, many of which, I have learned, have no definitive answers. However, I cherish the way art can provide alternative possibilities for clarity, for improved seeing and enhanced understanding of our own subjectivity. Allows us to discover how life circumstances such as love and loss can infiltrate our bodies. And lets us connect the outside to deep within us in pursuit of personal healing and daily health.

Arts in healthcare, while developing into an international multi-disciplinary field, continues to ponder its nomenclature: should we call it arts in medicine, or arts and health, or arts and wellness, or arts and medicine? Most recently, arts in health has emerged as the frequently used term for the field "dedicated to using the power of the arts to enhance human health and wellbeing."[79] Another more dynamic phrasing also being suggested is arts for healing, implying that "healing" carries much more emotional weight than "health." One day, perhaps, we will experience the arts as medicine. Your doctor delivers your prescription order: write a poem or make a dance every day. The field's naming has been as elusive as its self-identification—complementary, holistic, integrative—amidst a western tradition that initially resisted its legitimacy.

Beyond the challenges of naming and definition, we have seen firsthand how the arts can reconnect professional caregivers to themselves. In a workplace that requires the constant care of others, creative expression provides a much-needed respite for caregivers' self-care. Invoking creative expression has been shown to reduce everyday anxieties and stress while helping with depression.[80] Evidence reveals that engaging in artistic activities can enhance one's mood, emotions and other psychological states as well as impact heart rate, blood pressure, and other physiological parameters.[81] In some instances, according to the National Institute of Health, art making improves one's immune system while helping with the burden of chronic disease.

Arts in health continues to extend its reach organized around six core areas of specialization—healthcare environments, patient experiences, clinical services, the care of caregivers, health science education, and community health and well-being. These six focus areas are joined in a common mission to support health as defined by the World Health Organization (WHO)—"a state of complete physical, mental, and social well-being and not merely the absence of disease or infirmity."[82] In a range of public sectors including medicine, public health and community development, the arts are being implemented to inspire, educate and heal. Research in the U.S. and elsewhere continues to document the arts' impact on health while being extolled by distinguished health experts such as Vivek H. Murthy (MD, MBA), the 19th Surgeon General of the United States. "Within the arts lies a powerful but largely untapped force for healing. The arts and sciences are two sides of the same coin, which is our shared humanity."[83] Dr. Murthy opines that one's ability to live a fulfilled, healthy life depends on ways to bring the arts and sciences together.

Our work and that of other artists will surely continue to expand the relationship between the arts and healing. In tandem with research exploring the question of how creativity functions in the brain, the field of arts and personal wellness continues to develop at a rapid pace. Partnering with caregivers has revealed to us the connectivity between creative expression and healing. The future will inevitably uncover more about how the arts can continue to heal our caregivers, professional and personal—and all of us.

My publisher greenlighted this book a few weeks after Covid-19 was declared a pandemic. How ironic, again, that a creative act would speak about—predict—what was about to unfold throughout the world. Caregivers, risking their lives in unprecedented ways, to save some while protecting others. It has been a particular honor to write about the community of caregivers at this moment in history.

Endnotes

1. Philip Roth, *Portnoy's Complaint* (New York, Random House, 1969), p. 69.

2. *Bialy* is a Yiddish word for a baked delicacy originating in the Polish city of Bialystock. It is often sold in bagel bakeries although it has a different shape—bialys have a depression in the center vs. the bagel's hole. Both are delicious with a schmear (smear) of cream cheese.

3. *Boone v. Coe* - In 1913, a beleaguered Kentucky farmer and his family left their home based on an oral promise given by a Texas landowner. The Kentucky farmer, enticed by the promise of a new home and fertile land, traveled 55 days, braving the elements, to discover that the Texan had changed his mind. While the facts depicted gross hardships and loss for the farmer, the law was not on his side—don't count on anyone's promise unless there is a written agreement.

4. Martha Myers, *Don't Sit Down, The Life and Work of Martha Myers* (New York, 2018), p. 3.

5. www.stuartpimsler.com is our company website that contains examples and vimeo links to many of the performance works and caregiving workshops mentioned throughout this book.

6. Susanne K. Langer, *The Magic Circle, in Feeling And Form: A Theory Of Art* (New York, Charles Scribner's Sons, 1953), p. 191. Accessed March 29, 2019 from http://archive.org/details/LangerSusanneKFeelingAndFormATheoryOfArt1953.

7. In 1993, after being interviewed by a writer for *The Toronto Sun* about a workshop Suzanne and I had conducted at an area treatment center, we named our work *Caring for the Caregiver*. In the 25 years since, this moniker has been used by many in the arts-in-health field. However, it continues to be the name of our program that we have presented throughout the U.S. and abroad.

8. Anatole Broyard, "The patient examines the doctor" (chapter 3) in *Intoxicated by My Illness: And Other Writings on Life and Death*, ed. Alexandra Broyard (New York: Fawcett Columbine, 1992), p. 57. Accessed March 17, 2019 from http://www.masshumanities.org/files/programs/LitMed/readings/Broyard_Anatole_The_Patient_Examines_the_Doctor.pdf

9. Ibid, foreword, p. xiv.

10. Bliss Broyard, *One Drop, My Father's Hidden Life–A Story of Race and Hidden Secrets* (New York, Back Bay Books, 2007), pp. 12, 474.

11. Anatole Broyard (1992), p. 54.

12. Bruce W. Newton et al., Is there hardening of the heart during medical school?, *Academic Medicine* 83, no. 3 (March 2008), 244–249. Accessed May 26, 2021 from https://doi.org/10.1097/ACM.0b013e3181637837.

13. Mohammadreza Hojat et. al., The devil is in the third year: a longitudinal study of erosion of empathy in medical school, *Academic Medicine* 84, no. 9 (September 2009). Accessed November 11, 2020 from https://pubmed.ncbi.nlm.nih.gov/19707055/

14. Melanie Neumann et al., Empathy decline and its reasons: a systematic review of studies with medical students and residents, *Academic Medicine* 86, no. 8 (August 2011), 996–1009. Accessed May 26, 2021 from https://doi.org/10.1097/ACM.0b013e318221e615.

15. Ibid, p. 12.

16. Newton et al, Ibid.

17. Jessica Freedman, 5 questions, answers about attending osteopathic medical school (medical school admissions doctor) *US News*, December 16, 2014. Accessed September 18, 2020 from https://www.usnews.com/education/blogs/medical-school-admissions-doctor/2014/12/16/5-qustions-answers-about-attending-osteopathic-medical-school.

18. Troy Parks, Report reveals severity of burnout by specialty, *AMA Wire*, January 31, 2017. Accessed September 19, 2020 from https://wire.ama-assn.org/life-career/report-reveals-severity-burnout-specialty.

19. The Institute of American Stress, Compassion fatigue (2020). Accessed September 20, 2020 from http://www.stress.org/military/for-practitionersleaders/compassion-fatigue/

20. Parks, Ibid.

21. Suzanne Costello & Stuart Pimsler (2015), *Transforming the Doctor-Patient Relationship*, Student Response/Evaluation, Michigan State University College of Osteopathy.

22. Eric J. Cassell, Illness and disease, *The Hastings Center Rep.* 6, no. 2 (Apr. 1976), 27-37.

23. Michael Specter, Public nuisance. *The New Yorker*, 2002, p. 43.

24. Ibid, p. 42.

25. Ibid, p. 42.

26. Michael Millenson, *Demanding Medical Excellence: Doctors and Accountability in the Information Age* (Chicago: The University of Chicago Press, 1997), p. 316.

27. EULAR Recommendations, Education for people with inflammatory arthritis (December 1, 2017). Accessed January 18, 2021 from https://www.eular.org/search.cfm

28. Raffi Khatchadourian, How to control a machine with your brain, *The New Yorker*, November 26, 2018. Accessed December 13, 2020 from https://www.newyorker.com/magazine/2018/11/26/how-to-control-a-machine-with-your-brain

29. Judith Orloff M.D., *The Power of Surrender* (New York, Harmony, 2014), p. 100.

30. Kerri L. Johnson and Maggie Shiffrar, eds., *People Watching: Social, Perceptual, and Neurophysiological Studies of Body Perception* (New York: Oxford University Press, 2013), p. 3.

31. Hanan Parvez, Body language: crossing the arms, *PsychMechanics*, 2018. Accessed March 30, 2020 from https://www.psychmechanics.com/2015/04/body-language-crossing-arms.html.

32. Judith Lynne Hanna, *Dancing to Learn-The Brain's Cognition, Emotion and Movement* (Maryland, Rowan & Littlefield, 2015), p. 17.

33. Ibid.

34. Kimerer L. LaMothe, *Why We Dance: A Philosophy of Bodily Becoming* (New York, Columbia University Press, 2015), p. 5.

35. Anna Halprin, *Dance as a Healing Art: Returning to Health with Movement and Imagery* (Mendocino, CA: LifeRhythm Books, 2000), p. 13.

36. Ibid, p. 15.

37. Alice W. Flaherty, Performing the art of medicine, *Total Art Journal* 1, no. 1 (Summer 2011). Accessed May 28, 2019 from http://totalartjournal. com/wp-content/uploads/2011/08/Flaherty_PerformingTheArtOfMedicine_ TotalArtJournal_Vol.1_No.1_Summer2011.pdf.

38. LaMothe, Ibid.

39. John Ratey with Eric Hagerman, *Spark: The Revolutionary New Science of Exercise and the Brain* (New York: Little, Brown & Company, 2008), p. 56.

40. www.stuartpimsler.com

41. Langer, Ibid, p. 191.

42. Leeat Granek, Grief in health care professionals: when screening for major depression is needed—reply. *Archives of Internal Medicine*, 172, no. 22 (December 10, 2012), 1768-1769.

43. Ibid, p. 1768.

44. Ibid, p. 1769.

45. Naomi Rachel Remen, *Kitchen Table Wisdom - Stories That Heal* (New York: Penguin Group, 1996), p. 52.

46. Ibid, p. 52.

47. Anatole Broyard, Ibid, pp. 33-58.

48. Alice W. Flaherty, Performing the art of medicine, *Total Art Journal* 1, no. 1 (Summer 2011). Accessed May 28, 2019 from http://totalartjournal. com/wp-content/uploads/2011/08/Flaherty_PerformingTheArtOfMedicine_ TotalArtJournal_Vol.1_No.1_Summer2011.pdf

49. Ella Al-Shamahi, *The Handshake: A Gripping History* (Great Britain, Profile Books, 2021), p. 2.

50. Solrun Brenk Rønning & Stål Bjørkly, The use of clinical role-play and reflection in learning therapeutic communication skills in mental health education: an integrative review, *Advances in Medical Education and Practice*, 10 (June 2019). Accessed July 26, 2017 from https://pubmed.ncbi.nlm. nih.gov/31417328/

51. Horst Hammitzsch, *Zen in the Art of the Tea Ceremony: A Guide to the Tea Way* (New York: St. Martin's Press, 1980), p. 46.

52. Kim Leddy, Dancing doctors, *Columbus Alive*, December 13, 1996, p. 9.

53. *Simcha* is a Yiddish word meaning joy.

54. Thomas Kirsch, What happens if health-care workers stop showing up? *The Atlantic*, March 24, 2020. Accessed May 28, 2020 from https://www. theatlantic.com/ideas/archive/2020/03/were-failing-doctors/608662/

55. Dawei Wang, Bo Hu, and Chang Hu, Clinical characteristics of 138 hospitalized patients with 2019 novel coronavirus–infected pneumonia in Wuhan, China, (February 2020). Accessed December 23, 2020 from https:// jamanetwork.com/journals/jama/fullarticle/2761044

56. Zahra Hirji, Thousands of US health care workers have been infected by the coronavirus. This is how each state stacks up, *BuzzFeed News*, April 9, 2020. Accessed May 26, 2020 from https://www.buzzfeednews.com/article/zahrahirji/us-health-care-workers-coronavirus

57. Elizabeth Cohen and Dr. Minali Nigam, CDC estimates more than 9,200 healthcare workers have been infected with Covid-19, *CNN*, April 15, 2020. Accessed May 16, 2020 from https://www.cnn.com/2020/04/15/health/coronavirus-9200-health-workers-infected/index.html

58. Bart Ehrman, Heaven and hell are not what Jesus preached, interview by Terry Gross, March 31, 2020. Accessed June 26, 2020 from https://www.npr.org/2020/03/31/824479587/heaven-and-hell-are-not-what-jesus-preached-religion-scholar-says

59. Paradise polled: Americans and the afterlife, *The Roper Center for Public Opinion Research*. Accessed June 26, 2020 from https://ropercenter.cornell.edu/paradise-polled-americans-and-afterlife

60. Simcha Paul Rafael, *Jewish Views of the Afterlife* (Lanham: Rowman & Littlefield, 2019), p. 159.

61. Alfonso Ortiz, *The Tewa World* (Chicago: University of Chicago Press, 1969), p. 50.

62. Thomas Lynch, *The Undertaking: Life Studies from the Dismal Trade* (New York: Penguin Group, 1997), p. 21.

63. Camille LeFevre, Life after loss, *Minneapolis Star Tribune*, January 26, 2001, p. 13.

64. Kay Harvey, Dancing with death, *Pioneer Press,* January 23, 2001, p. 5.

65. Ibid, p. 5.

66. Mark Strand, *Dark Harbor* (New York: Knopf Doubleday Publishing Group, 1994), p. 18.

67. Stuart Pimsler, Journal excerpt, November 15,1997.

68. Arlene Goldbard, Postscript to the past: notes toward a history of community arts. *High Performance* 64 (Winter, 1993). Accessed March 17, 2021 from http://www.darkmatterarchives.net/wp-content/uploads/2011/11/GoldbergCETAsanfrancisco.pdf

69. Goldbard, Ibid.

70. *Moving Inquiries* was created with Twin Cities hospice caregivers and SPDT artists. It was presented May 25-27, 2000 in the Weisman Art Museum galleries. The exhibit *Hospice: A Photographic Inquiry,* organized by the Corcoran Gallery of Art, was on view at the Weisman and served as a meaningful setting for *Moving Inquiries.*

71. The Society for the Arts in Healthcare was reorganized into the National Organization for Arts in Health (NOAH) in 2016 (thenoah.net)

72. Jill Sonke, Rusti Brandman, Judy Rollins, John Graham-Pole, The state of the arts in healthcare in the U.S., *Arts & Health* (September, 2009), p. 114.

73. Ibid.

74. Alexis Soloski, Jonathan Majors on *Lovecraft Country*: horror as a full body scream, *NY Times*, August 10, 2020. Accessed September 1, 2020 from https://www.nytimes.com/2020/08/13/arts/television/lovecraft-country-review.html

75. Columbia University Department of Neurology, *The History of Stroke,* 2015. Accessed October 26, 2017 from https://www.columbianeurology.org/neurology/staywell/document.php?id=33434#:~:text=History%20of%20Stroke,and%20change%20in%20well%2Dbeing.

76. Gabriela Rodriguez Gomez, *Re-Conceptualizing Social Medicine in Diego Rivera's History of Medicine in Mexico: The People's Demand for Better Health Mural.* University of California, 2012.

77. *LISTEN/Stories of Cancer and Resilience,* Twin Cities Public Television. Accessed May 26, 2021 from http://www.stuartpimsler.com/arts-healthcare/community-inclusive-projects

78. Sigrid Nunez, *The Friend* (New York, Riverhead Books, 2018), p. 164.

79. National Organization for Arts in Health. (2017). Arts, health, and well-being in America. San Diego, CA, p. 5.

80. Heather L. Stuckey DEd and Jeremy Nobel MD, The connection between art, healing and public health, *American Journal of Public Health,* (2010), 254-263.

81. R Staricoff and S Loppert, *Integrating the Arts into Health Care: Can We Affect Clinical Outcomes?* London: Royal College of Physicians, 2003.

82. National Organization for Arts in Health, Ibid, p. 5.

83. Ibid, p.1.

Acknowledgments

For the thousands of caregivers we have engaged—"super heroes in humble attire"—my gratitude for inviting Suzanne and me into your workplaces. Without your generosity of spirit, this book would not have been possible.

Our children, Sophia and Gabriel, fill me with joy every day. Thank you so much for your love and support and for reading the manuscript with much enthusiasm. I adore you!

My appreciation to my brother Randy for his love as well as other Pimsler and Kaizer family members, including my parents Cecile and Lenny. Thanks to Harry and Doris Costello who were enthusiastic champions of our work.

My artistic career has been realized in three different cities—New York, Columbus, Ohio, and Minneapolis, Minnesota. In each location, I have been fortunate to have friends, teachers and colleagues who have listened, questioned, laughed and supported me from the beginning. Thanks to Howard Bell, Kathy Burkman, Carolelinda Dickey, Liz Engelman, Jon Garness, Michael Howett, Ron Kajiwara, Michael Kasper, Pat Mahoney, Martha Myers, Daniel Nagrin, Karin Olson, Paul Virtucio and Steve Vogel.

Thank you "for your beautiful dancing" to all of the Stuart Pimsler Dance & Theater artists who dedicated themselves to our work over the years including Kurt Blomberg, Brian Evans, Susan Hamilton, Matt Jenson, Heather Klopchin, Kari Mosel, Janet Parrott, Stephen Patterson, Jesse Neumann-Peterson, Jennifer Pray, Nancy Wanich-Romita, Tiyo Siyolo, Scott Stafford, Laura Selle-Virtucio, Vanessa Voskuil, Roxane Wallace, the "Red Dancers" and all of our guest artists from across the globe.

This book has evolved over many years and my thanks to those who have helped it along: Sophia Diehl, Hannah Kramer, Kathleen Pender and editor, Elizabeth Zimmer. And Robin Brooks—friend, colleague and almost family—thank you!

The workshops, residencies, and performance works described in these pages have been presented by colleges, universities, performing arts centers hospitals, hospices, social service organizations, and other healthcare venues in the United States and abroad—thank you for inviting us to share our work with your communities.

I am greatly appreciative of the support for our arts in health endeavors over the years including the National Endowment for the Arts, Minnesota State Arts Board, McKnight Foundation, Metropolitan Regional Arts Council, Target, The Ohio Arts Council, the Greater Columbus Arts Council, the Lila Wallace Readers Digest Fund, the National Performance Network and individual Friends of Stuart Pimsler Dance & Theater.

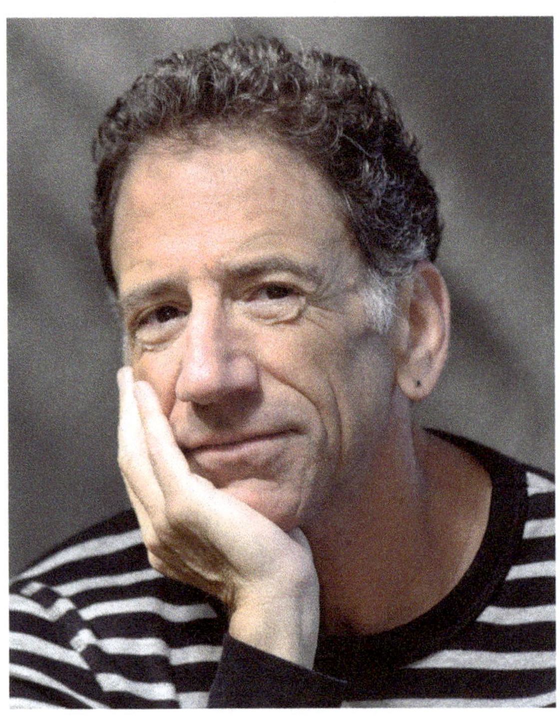

Photo credit: V. Paul Virtucio

STUART PIMSLER is a writer, director, choreographer, performer, and founder of Stuart Pimsler Dance & Theater (SPDT). He and SPDT artistic co-director Suzanne Costello have been internationally recognized for their work and leadership in the field of arts and health for over three decades. Stuart has created more than fifty performance works for SPDT, written a play for children, *My Grandmother's Tchotchkes,* and recently adapted the short story, MATINEE, into an interdisciplinary stage work. He has been honored with fellowships from the National Endowment for the Arts, McKnight Foundation, Ohio Arts Council and commissions worldwide. Stuart lives in Minneapolis with his family.

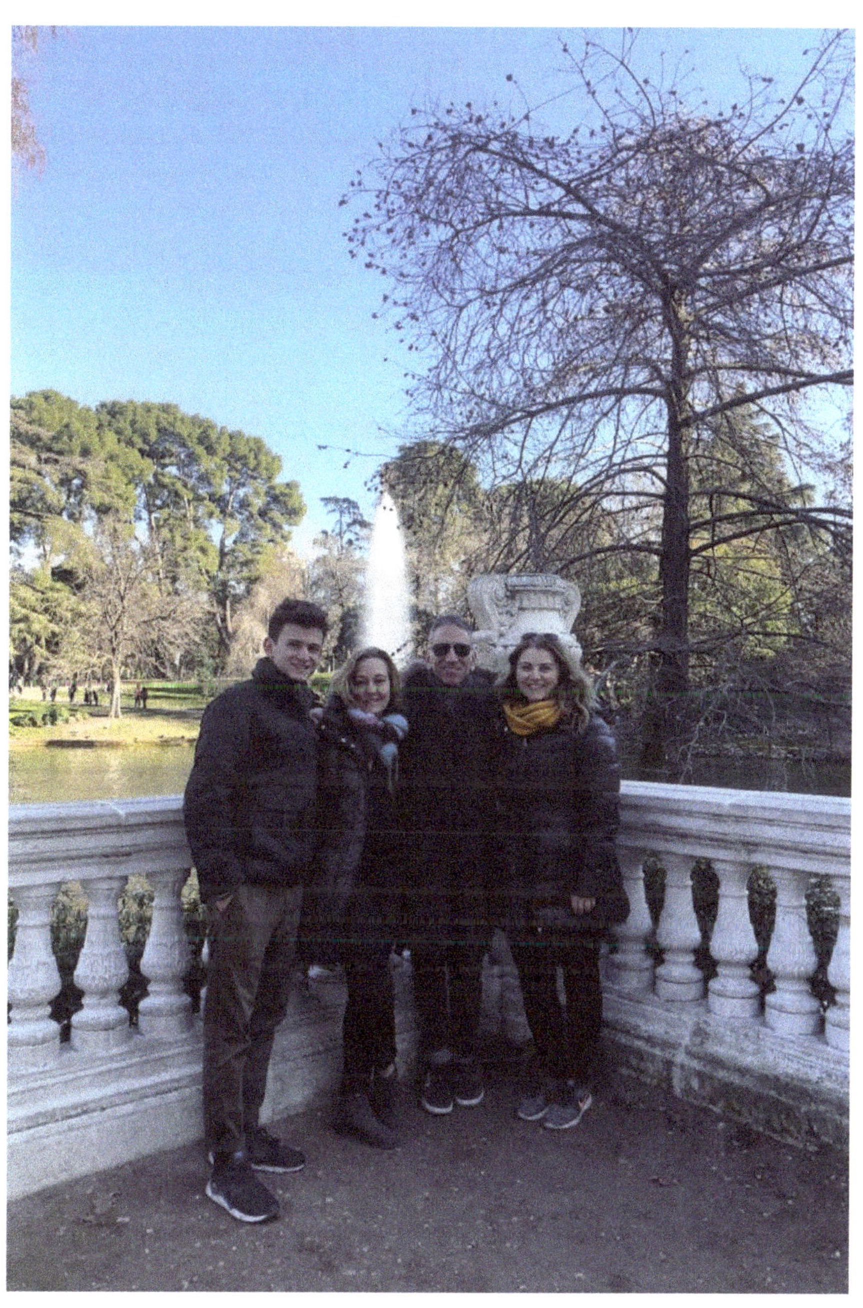

Gabe, Suzanne, Stuart & Sophia (2020)

www.ingramcontent.com/pod-product-compliance
Lightning Source LLC
Chambersburg PA
CBHW051125300726

48981CB00023B/554/J